A TIME TO ALIGN:

An Anusara® Yoga
Prenatal Guide for
Teachers, Students,
and New Moms

First Edition

by Sue Elkind
snlivingyoga.com
email: snyoga@mac.com

Cover photo: Art Streiber/AUGUST
Yoga illustrations: Sue Elkind
Book layout: Lynnell Koser & Sue Elkind
Editing: Dana Covello

Note: It is advisable for all pregnant women to consult with their physician before undertaking any
exercise program. This book is not intended as a substitute for professional medical care.

For my husband, Naime Jezzeny who teaches me everyday the importance of being true to oneself, and our two boys Luca and Milo who through my pregnancies ignited my passion for prenatal yoga.

This guide is the genesis of many prenatal offerings to come. It is Anusara's intention to fully serve the community from the heart in this way. The rapidly expanding need for prenatal Anusara yoga guidance will continue to inspire the subject's growth and expansion. — Anusara, Inc

This workbook is a labor of love, one that Sue has put together over the past ten years. Her vibrancy, well-honed teaching skills, and sensitivity to individual needs are earmarks of Sue's teaching — and ones that captured my heart as her student of yoga.

The information in this book is the result of passionate research and practical applications with pregnant women throughout the world as well as intensely personal observations based on her own experiences of pregnancy with her beloved sons, Luca and Milo.

Dr. Mae Sakharov, Ed. D
Educational consultant to ABC "20/20"

Anusara Yoga Invocation*

OM
Namah Shivaya Gurave
Satchidananda Murtaye
Nishprapanchaya Shantaya
Niralambaya Tejase

Translation:

I honor the essence of Being, the Auspicious One,

The luminous Teacher within and without,

Who assumes the forms of Truth,

Consciousness, and Bliss,

Is never absent, full of peace,

Ultimately free and sparkles with a divine luster.

* Chanting is a beautiful way to connect
mother and baby throughout pregnancy — the baby
delights in hearing the mother's voice.

This invocation can be offered as a prenatal lullaby
and often has a calming effect on the baby after birth.

TABLE OF CONTENTS

FOREWORD

Yoga invites us to engage deeply, to create connections, and to affirm wholly the fullness of our lives. And what gift in life presents a greater opportunity for yoga or a more profound offering of Grace than the experience of pregnancy?

The tradition of women caring for women extends deeply into the ancient yogas, and in Tantra we learn of the woman-sage Lopamudra. Lopamudra is the guardian of the life-giving inner waters; the presence of Grace holding purity within; and the teacher of midwives, yoginis, and all who seek the subtle powers of the Shakti's most receptive energies during prenatal care. Tradition says that Lopamudra was a princess born as a boon to the King of Kavera granted to him by none other than grandfather Creator Brahma. After she was married to the great sage Agastya, the princess took the form of water within her husband's sacred vessel. Once Agastya asked his yogic student to carry this vessel, but he could not bear its weight. And so the water that was Lopamudra spilt, rushing forth as the river Kaveri. When King Kavera bathed in this now-famous south Indian river that began as none other than his daughter's own form, he experienced his own liberation. And so it is that all who step into Lopamudra's subtle presence as the life-holding waters are too born to experience their freedom. What a story! But with a little Tantric ingenuity, we can further savor its sweetness.

Lopamudra's name means the seal or imprint (*mudra*) of interruption or sometimes even injury (*lopa*). As a child grows in the womb so this gift "interrupts" the usual patterns of life and creates its own imprint from inside out. Giving birth is a perfect, blessed "injury" creating the most auspicious gift we might ever receive. In the meantime, a baby floats and swims in its mother, the sacred vessel, protected there by love through partnership, and with the help of the mother's companions, shares her yogic journey. When a child is ready to spill forth into the world, from the inner waters of grace, she or he will come to purify, to bless, and even to liberate all who have come before as well as those who follow. Every mother becomes Lopamudra, that vessel of the sacred, the waters within her being a gift of Grace to the emergent life she holds, and her yoga the process by which to engage fully in the offerings of pregnancy and birth.

With Sue Elkind as your guide and the principles of Anusara yoga to lead the way, I know you are in the best of hands to make or advise others in this journey. For pregnant women, with the practices of yoga, you will feel even more deeply the imprint of that precious soul you carry within as the expression of your body's grace. May these teachings of yoga inspire your heart and empower your body! May the ancient teachings become present, enriching, and real in your experience of pregnancy, birth, and motherhood! I know this book will be a gift and a blessing, nothing less than another form of Lopamudra spilling forth her blessings and teachings, for once again the ancient sage presents herself in your own experience of yoga. Jaya Lopamudra the Sage! Jaya Mataji, the Auspicious Mother!

Douglas Brooks
Bristol, New York

MY STORY

My interest in prenatal yoga developed shortly after I began teaching yoga in the early 1990's. During one of my first public classes, I encountered a pregnant student who was in obvious need of extra assistance. Trying not to panic, I instinctively gave her as many props as I could find to help her modify her practice and stayed close by to remind her to breathe! After the session, I called a seasoned prenatal yoga teacher and friend, Susan Swan, to consult about what I had done. First she assured me that I did not do anything wrong or harmful. She then offered me some useful advice based on her wisdom and personal experiences in pregnancy and prenatal yoga. From that first experience, I was truly inspired to see how yoga and the state of pregnancy were deeply connected. I continued to seek out prenatal trainings over the next several years, fortunate to be in Los Angeles where prenatal yoga was flourishing and great inspiration abundant, particularly Gurmukh Khalsa. What I found interesting was how different each prenatal yoga class was — depending on the teacher and their school of influence. When I became pregnant and decided to teach prenatal yoga, Anusara yoga became the synthesizer of the multitude of resources I had gathered and helped to inspire my own voice to bloom.

My hope with this book is that teachers, students, and others interested in the connection between pregnancy and yoga will gain a deeper understanding of the many gifts that prenatal yoga offers for pregnancy, birth, and subsequently for parenting. A teacher trained to work with the specific conditions of the pregnant body — including the ability to encourage a student to really trust in her experience, can greatly help to create a safe, healthy, and empowering prenatal yoga practice.

My greatest source of prenatal wisdom has undoubtedly come from having two very different pregnancies and birth experiences. Although both were homebirths, my first pregnancy was much more conventional than the second. Being cautious after already having had a miscarriage, I listened diligently to my doctor and the spiritual guidance of my cherished doula Anna Verwaal (a doula is often translated as "mother's mother" and is there to support the mother during the birth process). My beloved yoga teacher, John Friend, offered wonderful insight into my personal practice and the best gift of all — the blessing to be my own teacher and explore my pregnancy and practice from a deep inner wisdom.

While I initially thought a conventional hospital birth would be my route, about four weeks before my first son, Luca, was born, I found a new house more suitable to do a home birth and switched to a midwife. When the first real contractions started, I felt that I had prepared as best as possible. What I did not expect was that my labor would last thirty-two hours. I was fully dilated when my water finally broke in the bathtub. My midwife noticed the amniotic fluid contained meconium (a thick, tar-like stool that a baby typically releases after he or she is born). Luca had a bowel movement while still in the womb, which meant there was a chance he could aspirate meconium into his lungs upon arrival. Although this situation is fairly common, it was none-the-less frightening. Our pediatrician, Jay Gordon, came rushing to the house hoping to avoid taking Luca to the hospital. After listening to his lungs for a solid hour, everyone agreed it was not worth the risk. Luca spent the first week of his life in neo-natal intensive care with tubes up his nose to help him breathe and had continuous monitoring for infection. Looking back, Luca and I had extraordinary moments together the first hour of his life, and I was fortunate to avoid the higher risk of a c-section surgery, a standard procedure when meconium is detected. Even though my home birth did not go according to my plan, I had an important revelation: birth is not just about a mother's wishes and plans. Luca's birth wasn't just my dance.

My second son, Milo, on the other hand, arrived while I was in a very deep state of meditation — without even pushing — in a truly bucolic birth in the comforts of our dimly lit bedroom. Both my husband Naime and I were astonished at the beauty and bliss of Milo's sweet entrance into the world and bathed for hours in the afterglow. Reflecting on this pregnancy, I barely had any intervention, choosing instead to use a stethoscope when possible and the skillful hands of my midwives, Shelly Girard and Seannie Gibson. I stayed 'tuned in' through regular meditation and trusted what I heard inwardly with even greater sensitivity and awareness. My confidence to do this was bolstered immensely by having both the strength and support of my midwives who continuously guided me, along with my family and friends standing close by.

Looking back at my birth experiences, I realize how important it is for a pregnant woman to be surrounded by loving, supportive, and understanding friends. Without the emotional security of a *kula* (community of like-minded hearts), it is much harder to relax and trust the wisdom that is inherently within. This is one of the main reasons why I feel prenatal yoga classes, if available, are such a powerful and indispensable part of a woman's pregnancy for both experienced practitioners and those new to yoga.

THE INNER WISDOM OF YOGA IN PREGNANCY

From one creative Universal force, all of life emerges. Divine energy takes the form of everything manifest and unseen — expanding, contracting, and radiating from this light of existence. Each one of us is an expression of this supreme consciousness, whose innate nature is love and joy. Yoga strengthens this awareness and enables us to step fully into ourselves — body, mind, and heart. As we learn to trust in this universal connection and recognize how deeply supported we are, we can more freely let go of fears and experience our lives with greater understanding, compassion, and joy.

Pregnancy offers a woman the opportunity to tap into and participate in the creative energy of the Universe. The threshold into motherhood is an extremely powerful time of heightened sensitivity and growth on multiple levels. From a yogic perspective, pregnancy is a sacred time for a woman to discover her own intuitive strength and nurture the creative feminine power within. For many women, this inner shift of awareness occurs naturally. Instinctually, the body lures the mind inward to notice and care for all the physical, emotional, and hormonal changes beginning to occur. As the fetus begins to grow, a powerful maternal urge to nurture and protect often naturally ignites. Practicing yoga enhances and empowers a woman's experience of pregnancy and birth on all levels — physically, emotionally, and spiritually. Through the ever-unfolding gifts of yoga, the process of giving birth becomes not only an invitation to deepen one's innermost connection to the Universe but also a celebration of the profound, regenerative, and sacred power each woman holds.

Pregnancy and birth are both singularly extraordinary and universally common. Everyone alive on this planet is united in the commonality that they must be 'born' to get here — yet throughout the world, birth experiences range from the most primitive and natural, to the most scheduled and scientific. We are both cultural and natural beings, regardless of how we arrived on this planet. The power to think and reason does not make us any less connected to nature — although sometimes it is our own minds that get in the way of that understanding. Practicing yoga while pregnant invites a woman to pulsate between her natural and cultural sides. Some women more easily recognize the cultured side of pregnancy — embracing their noted glow and outer beauty. However it is equally essential for a pregnant woman to draw into her innermost primal essence — not only as a means to uncover and transform any deep-seated fears but also to strengthen her resolve and recognize that the power to create life is inherent. Through the process of diving inward, a woman can experience her divine nature more authentically, allowing her to see more beauty and interconnectedness in the world.

When a woman has the courage to face the darkness of her pregnancy head on, she discovers that beneath the fear and discomfort is the support of the primordial Goddess, Kali. Often depicted as pure blackness, Kali is the first Hindu Goddess to take form. She is sometimes known as original mother, though she is nothing like you would expect a mother to be! She is radical, wild, and ferocious, and while she loves to stretch us to our outer boundaries, her intention is always to take us deeper into our hearts to feel her unconditional love. When a woman is going through labor, she must learn to trust her own Kali-like nature and release any inhibitions around her pregnancy and the process of giving birth. If she is able step fully into her experience, before accepting or denying it, she will feel the nurturing roar of Kali and discover even more strength available within her — empowering her birth and preparing her for motherhood. It is also the embrace of Kali that allows a woman to move forward when her labor takes an unplanned course.

The pulsation of pregnancy also calls for a woman to seek the wisdom and generosity of others and to appreciate the beauty of her outer environment. All of the many ways a woman can enjoy and share her pregnancy with the world are reflected in the refined, cultured energy of the Goddess Shri. She becomes the expression of all that is beautiful and sacred about being pregnant. A woman taps into Shri when she chooses to listen to her body each day and comes from a place of love, honor, and respect for herself and the miracle of life growing within.

In addition to connecting to the power and the beauty of the goddess within, it is helpful for a pregnant woman to remember she is not alone in the birth process. It benefits a woman greatly to surround herself with a competent and loving team of support so she can relax and trust them to guide her to the safest delivery possible. In particular just being in the company of other pregnant women in prenatal yoga classes may create an instant sense of community — a place for information, understanding, and friendship.

PLANNING FOR PREGNANCY

There's a funny thing that happens to many women somewhere between their mid 20's, 30's, and 40's. Thoughts may begin to creep in about babies, and as much as the modern woman wants to deny them, the urge is strong. In many ways, it is the most natural instinct a woman can have. It's hormonal. It's evolutionary. Once the seed is planted, every thought begins to water that idea into more possibility — and ultimately, for some, into motherhood.

A woman enters her pregnancy in myriad ways. Whether it is planned and conventional, unconventional or unexpected, Mother Nature has no 'moral' preference regarding conception. The simple, yet complex scientific dance of sperm penetrating egg has yielded results for eons. While a woman cannot control the intricacies during that time of conception or her pregnancy, there are some helpful things she can do beforehand to ensure a healthier experience from preconception through childbirth.

The first thing she can do is slow down and examine her current life. If work responsibilities are piling up and each day ends in stress, adding a child to the mix isn't going to make it easier. As hard as it may be, creating more space now, before pregnancy, is an important step in preparing for motherhood — physically, mentally, and emotionally. During both of my pregnancies, I found taking regular walks in nature and routinely having nourishing, romantic meals with Naime helped to alleviate stress and restore deeper commitments to creating a family.

Good physical health should be a priority before conceiving. Getting a thorough doctor's examination, for both the woman and man, can help detect and/or ward off any unwanted problems or conditions (i.e checking health of sperm, screening for sexually transmitted diseases). A woman should find an OB/GYN with whom she is comfortable and have a full check-up including a pap smear and blood work. With her doctor's advice, she may consider taking prenatal supplements (including folic acid to prevent neural tube defects) and start paying closer attention to her diet. I recommend buying organic food and avoiding chemicals, pesticides, and genetically modified foods as much as possible, as well as drinking filtered water to avoid lead, excess chlorine, metals, and synthetic hormones. To improve her overall health and in preparation for the extra resources needed for the healthy development of a baby, a woman can increase certain foods such as organic fresh produce; whole grain foods; organic chicken, fish, and eggs; and natural live yogurt. Fortunately, there are many books and web sites that offer nutrition for preconception and pregnancy as well as ways to maintain a healthy balanced diet for life (see the Additional Resources section beginning on page 78).

A consistent yoga practice prior to conception will help cultivate a deeper sense of awareness and attune a woman's body to its natural rhythms. It also will strengthen and open the body, preparing it for childbirth. Yoga time should include breath work and meditation. Using visualizations of pregnancy and motherhood can help... energy follows intention.

It is important for a woman to remember there is no 'right' way to be pregnant or to give birth. Just as each person is unique in their own way, so too is every pregnancy unique, deeply personal, and cloaked in majesty. Yoga teaches us to celebrate both our diversity and commonality. It invites us to affirm the particular way in which the Divine has taken form as our individual experience and the universal process of childbirth. Oftentimes, a woman feels she has failed if her ideas around getting pregnant or even childbirth do not go according to her plan. Yoga teaches a woman to let go of expectations and to remember the baby too is part of the process and may have a different plan.

PREGNANCY HURDLES: MISCARRIAGE AND INFERTILITY

I can honestly say that I never had the urge to have a baby before getting pregnant. The closest I had come to that mothering instinct was 'birthing' a new yoga studio in Los Angeles, which I poured my heart and soul into making happen. To my surprise, only weeks into the studio opening, Naime and I discovered we were going to have a 'real' baby. I felt overwhelmed to say the least. When we finally both got over the shock and we contemplated our future together as a family, we actually discovered a deep joy arising. Then, almost nine weeks into the pregnancy, I had a miscarriage. It was more of a shocker than getting pregnant. Being a health-conscious yoga teacher, the possibility never entered my mind. We grieved the loss, as expected, but also recognized the spark was still present within us. The seed had been planted, so to speak, and we felt a definite shift into a deeper commitment to our relationship. I owe so much of my recovery from miscarriage to my regular yoga and meditation practice. Asana helped me to physically regain strength more efficiently, while meditation aided my emotional state — helping me stay connected to the little soul I knew would still someday join us.

We spent the next twelve months 'keeping the door open' — with the intention to get pregnant with grace and ease. I kept my prenatal supplements going with the doctor's advice and visualized our family in my meditations. We decided to get married and shortly after, to our sweet delight, discovered we were pregnant. We were infinitely more prepared for our pregnancy having that year between miscarriage and conception. Although it doesn't always work out that way, for us having that time helped us more fully 'conceive' the life we wanted to create.

Miscarriage is always a possibility, particularly in early stages of pregnancy. That is why during the first trimester some women choose to contain the news of the secret life growing within. Fifteen percent of known pregnancies end in miscarriage, according to the American College of Obstetricians and Gynecologists (ACOG), and the majority of them happen in the first trimester. When a woman discovers she's had a miscarriage, it is often wrought with feelings of guilt as she wonders what she might have done to cause it. The majority of the time, it is just the way Mother Nature corrects herself. Grieving the loss of the fetus is healthy and important, and may create an even greater certainty within a woman about her desire to become a mother. There have been many cases of healthy births after even as many as four miscarriages beforehand.

The recovery after a miscarriage is different for every woman. In general, the later the pregnancy loss, the greater the period of physical recovery. Whether a woman miscarries naturally or surgically by dilation and curettage (D&C) may also impact the healing process. The latter (surgically) takes a considerably shorter time to recover from — averaging around two weeks for bleeding to fully subside and hormone-induced mood swings to even out. Early pregnancy miscarriage resembles light to heavy menstrual bleeding and cramps, which is why some women do not realize they are having one. I recommend waiting until after all heavy bleeding has stopped before a woman returns to her regular yoga practice (as well as getting approval from her doctor). She should also avoid ALL inversions (even Down Dog) until she has completely recovered. There are some helpful yoga poses to do at home that may provide relief from cramping and mood swings. Seated forward bends like Upavista Konasana and reclining gentle twists, both with a bolster propped up underneath the belly, may provide comfort.

The emotional recovery is another story altogether and could take substantially longer, especially considering no two people grieve in the same way. *Pranayama* (see the breathing exercises beginning on page 33) and meditation are both helpful tools in supporting a woman throughout her personal journey towards healing. A regular yoga routine, once the physical body has recovered, will also help to keep her energy levels up and gradually uplift her spirits.

The following is a list of contemplations and affirmations to include in a meditation practice in the event of a miscarriage:

'I understand this was just Mother Nature's way, and I am not at fault.'
'I am hopeful the perfect soul will be back again soon.'
'My body is healing as it should and has the wisdom to create life.'
'I trust that all is well and happening in its perfect time.'

If a couple is having difficulty conceiving, both parties should seek medical attention to better understand what, if any, physical limitations are present. A woman should discontinue taking birth control pills (or remove her IUD, if applicable) for a solid three months before trying to conceive to give her body a chance to readjust and restore normal metabolic functions. Caffeine, alcohol, and smoking may increase the risk of miscarriage and birth defects and should be minimized or avoided. To ensure she is getting the necessary vitamins and minerals, a woman should consider taking prenatal vitamins (including folic acid), and if she is a strict vegetarian, consult with a nutritionist to make sure certain foods, like soy, are not affecting her fertility.

In addition to getting medical advice, a woman can try treating infertility using Anusara yoga's Universal Principles of Alignment (for more information on infertility refer to the article by Anusara yoga founder John Friend in Timothy McCall's book *Yoga as Medicine: The Yogic Prescription for Health and Healing*). The first thing an experienced yoga teacher should look for is whether a woman's energy is 'up-rooted'. Stress, of any kind, is a big reason for this disruption in the natural, downward flow of energy (*apana vayu*). Overworking, excessively wearing high heels, or even losing touch with one's 'softer' feminine side, can all cause this type of aggravation. Depending on where a woman holds her stress, her legs, pelvis, and/or back muscles can over tighten and actually cause a lift or shift in the inner organs — including the ovaries. Once the ovaries are even slightly agitated, a woman's ability to conceive may become greatly reduced.

The femurs (upper leg bones) will usually shift forward in the hip socket with this type of disruption of *apana vayu*. A simple way to check a woman's state is to look at her legs while she's lying down on the floor (on her back with her legs straight.) If her legs are lifted up away from the floor (even when you actively have her move them down) the femurs are too far forward. While supine, rooting the femur bones down (towards the hamstrings) will help to re-align the energy flows and optimally align the inner organs. Using the principles of Anusara yoga, a woman with uprooted femurs should emphasize Inner Spiral™ in all her poses — making sure she turns the inner edges of her feet, legs, and pelvis 'in', moves them 'back', and even widens them 'apart' before scooping her tailbone (for more details on Inner Spiral, see the next chapter: An Introduction to Anusara Yoga). The infertility yoga sequence beginning on page 72 focuses on the poses and principles to help those who may experience difficulty conceiving.

AN INTRODUCTION TO ANUSARA YOGA

One of the first things I learned as an Anusara yoga teacher was to look for the beauty in my students before adjusting their posture. I was trained to see the body as a 'temple that houses the Divine' and to make physical, therapeutic adjustments to enhance the light that was already present. This life-affirming attitude continues to inspire every aspect of my teaching and helps to set the tone in my classes for students to step more fully into their hearts. When I began to teach prenatal yoga, it was seamless how complementary this philosophy was to pregnancy and how truly supportive the Universal Principles of Alignment are in allowing a woman to more confidently step into her potential and relieve her aches and pains.

The Sanskrit word *anusara* (a-nu-sar-a) translates as "to be in the flow of Nature," "flowing with Grace," and "to follow your heart." Anusara yoga takes the premise that everything in life is the pulsation of Supreme Consciousness (Shiva), who has taken form as all things manifest (Shakti). The body and the mind are honored as sacred vessels through which we can discover our true nature and celebrate our lives as a gift of Grace.

Anusara yoga incorporates Universal Principles of Alignment with a life-affirming Shiva-Shakti Tantric-based yogic philosophy of intrinsic Goodness. It seeks to optimally align the body, mind, and spirit and invites us to step more fully into our potential and with the flow of Life itself. Anusara yoga is an all-inclusive yoga that welcomes diversity and encourages everyone to see the world as Shri   full of beauty, abundance, and value. In honoring the Divine in all beings, we accept the world and ourselves as we are and learn to respond from a place of love and trust.

THE THREE A'S™
OF ANUSARA YOGA

There are three A's (Attitude, Alignment, and Action™) that make up the foundation of Anusara yoga. When they are all performed fully, they help to optimize one's physical and spiritual experience of yoga.

Attitude is defined as the power of the heart's intention. It is the most powerful of the three A's, lighting the way as a force behind every action and expression. Attitude is the place from which a pregnant woman can begin to honor herself as a Goddess. It invites her to recognize the miracle of life growing within and reminds her to see the process of birth — in whatever form it takes — as Sacred.

Alignment refers to the way in which a pregnant woman optimally aligns her body using the Universal Principles of Alignment, how she chooses to infuse every movement with breath and love, and how she respects the process of pregnancy, doing what feels best on each day.

Action involves balancing the dynamic pulsation of Muscular Energy™ and Organic Energy™ to protect the natural tendencies of a pregnant body toward over-stretch or strain (see the next section on the Universal Principles of Alignment).

The three A's support the three trimesters by offering a woman tools to keep herself balanced and healthy throughout her pregnancy. During every trimester, contemplating Attitude is a way for a pregnant woman to honor her journey, regardless of how she may feel physically, spiritually, and emotionally on any given day. As her body changes, she can put her energy and strength into learning Alignment in order to keep her body feeling optimal. As she progresses from pregnancy into motherhood — particularly during her delivery and birth, she has the opportunity to put into Action all that she's learned.

The following is a list of prenatal contemplations for each of the A's of Anusara yoga:

ATTITUDE

DEFINITION: The power of the heart's intention.

PRENATAL CONTEMPLATION:

What qualities of the heart am I feeling today?

What is motivating me in my practice?

Am I able to see something beautiful in my pregnancy today?

What can I do to honor myself and the baby more today?

Am I open to whatever course my pregnancy and labor may take?

ALIGNMENT

DEFINITION: The mindful awareness of how all the parts of the self are connected.

PRENATAL CONTEMPLATION:

How is my body changing today?

How can I best support these changes?

Are my thoughts/emotions taking me into or out of alignment?

ACTION

DEFINITION: Participating with the natural energetic flow of the body that is both stabilizing (engaging) and freeing (expanding).

PRENATAL CONTEMPLATION:

Have I been using the right amount of effort in my practice today?

Have I spent time nurturing/taking care of myself?

Have I given proper attention to my growing baby?

Have I let others help me?

THE UNIVERSAL PRINCIPLES OF ALIGNMENT™ OF ANUSARA YOGA

The Universal Principles of Alignment are biomechanical principles that guide students to the optimal experience of their body, mind, and heart. They are organized into five energetic steps that pulsate sequentially between expanding and contracting, reflecting the Universal pulsation of life itself. For more details on these principles, I recommend getting the Anusara Yoga Teacher Training Manual or finding a trained Anusara yoga teacher in your area via anusara.com.

The five principles, which are to be done in sequential order, are:

1. Open to Grace™
2. Muscular Energy™
3. Inner Spiral™ (Expanding Spiral)
4. Outer Spiral™ (Contracting Spiral)
5. Organic Energy™

OPEN TO GRACE

The first Universal Principle of Alignment of Anusara yoga is the overarching principle that holds all the others. It helps us establish both the outer foundation of the pose and also inspires our inner intention. Opening to Grace is an invitation to experience the full possibility of our own self and our deepest connection to the Whole. This expansive quality of Opening to Grace can be felt by softening our edges and allowing our heart and inner body to naturally brighten from the inside out. The breath is a wonderful tool to help us experience this invitation of Grace and reflect on our highest intention of the practice.

It is important to remember that Grace is not something outside of us or something we must strive for or attain. Grace is ever-present within us and is experienced as the very presence of our own Self. Grace is truly a gift and in that way, we don't have to 'do' anything to receive Her — for She is the one breathing us. To experience the gift of Grace, take a few moments to soften inwardly and connect to the rhythm of your breath and the pulse of your heart. Allow yourself the opportunity to taste the invitation of Grace as the very energy that holds every thought, feeling, and form together.

MUSCULAR ENERGY

The second Universal Principle of Alignment in Anusara yoga is the stabilizing energy that draws us into and connects us to our core. It literally joins the different parts of our body, integrating the outer body (skin, muscles, and bones) to the radiant and expanded inner body.

There are three primary components to Muscular Energy:
1. Hug the muscles to the bones.
2. Hug into the midline.
3. Draw in from the periphery to the core.

The first component of Muscular Energy, 'hugging the muscles to the bones,' is a sweet and sensitive engagement (as opposed to gripping or hardening the muscles). The direction of energy moves from the skin to the muscles to the bones, resulting in an even tone on all sides of the body.

The second component, 'hugging to the midline,' is the movement of Muscular Energy from all directions to the vertical (midline) axis. For example, isometrically squeezing the legs towards each other is one way to create the engagement to the midline.

The third component, 'drawing in from the periphery to the core,' moves energy from the distal to the core (or proximal). For example, Muscular Energy in the legs in standing poses moves from the feet to the pelvic focal point.

INNER SPIRAL/EXPANDING SPIRAL

The third Universal Principle of Alignment, Inner Spiral, is an ever-expanding energy spiral that widens the back body in both the legs/hips and upper back/shoulders. It works in conjunction with the fourth Universal Principle of Alignment, Outer Spiral, to help to align the body and increase the flow of energy. Inner Spiral always precedes Outer Spiral.

There are three primary effects of Inner Spiral on the hips/legs:
1. Turns the front of the feet, legs, and pelvis inward toward the midline (IN).
2. Moves the inner edges of the feet, legs, and pelvis backward (BACK).
3. Broadens the legs and pelvis laterally apart (APART).

Inner Spiral of the shoulders/arms:
1. Expands the upper back and back of the shoulders.
2. Widens the shoulder blades away from each other.

In all arm planes, except when the arms are in the overhead plane, this action is created by internally rotating the arms. When the arms are in the overhead plane, this action is created by externally rotating the arms.

OUTER SPIRAL/CONTRACTING SPIRAL

The fourth Universal Principle of Alignment, Outer Spiral, is an ever-contracting energy spiral that draws inward toward the core and narrows the back body in both the hips/legs and upper back/shoulders. Inner Spiral and Outer Spiral harmoniously balance each other, helping to refine the energy flows in the body.

There are three primary effects of Outer Spiral on the hips/legs:
1. Turns the pelvis, legs, and feet outward (OUT).
2. Moves the inner edges of the pelvis (tailbone, base of sacrum, and sitting bones) forward (FORWARD).
3. Draws the sides of the pelvis and legs toward the midline (TOGETHER).

Outer Spiral of shoulders/arms:
1. Contracts the upper back and back of the shoulders.
2. Draws the shoulder blades towards each other.

In all arm planes, except when the arms are in the overhead plane, this action is created by externally rotating the arms. When the arms are in the overhead plane, this action is created by internally rotating the arms.

ORGANIC ENERGY

The last Universal Principle of Alignment, Organic Energy, is the complement to Muscular Energy. Muscular Energy stabilizes to the core, and Organic Energy expands energy away from the core.

Like Muscular Energy, there are three components to Organic Energy:
1. Extend from the core to the periphery.
2. Expand from the midline.
3. Expand concentrically from the bones out.

The first component of Organic Energy, 'extending from the core to the periphery,' moves energy from the core (proximal) to the distal. For example, in standing poses, organic energy in the legs moves from the pelvis (core) out through the feet (distal).

The second component, 'expanding from the midline,' laterally expands energy from the vertical axis out into all directions. For example, the legs and pelvis expand out from the midline of the body.

The third component, 'expanding concentrically from the bones,' is an energetic flow that moves from the bone to the muscles to the skin and beyond. For example, the legs and hips expand evenly on all sides of the bones.

A HEALTHY PREGNANCY WITH ANUSARA YOGA

Anusara yoga provides great support for a woman in all facets of her pregnancy. On the deepest level, it reminds her that the currents of Grace are always guiding her to be in her heart. On the physical level, the Universal Principles of Alignment work seamlessly to strengthen and align the body so a woman feels more comfortable and confident during her uncertain journey into birth and motherhood.

Opening to Grace serves all the trimesters of pregnancy by helping a woman stay present with what is happening inside (and out), remaining attuned to a Universal support. It reminds a woman to mindfully set her foundation, expand the breath into each pose and fill the inner body with bright intentions. This is particularly helpful as her center of gravity changes and balance becomes an issue. The expansive quality of Opening to Grace is especially important in the later days of pregnancy when the weight of the baby pulls a woman's belly forward. By breathing into her 'back body,' a woman supports her lower back from over arching and straining. Taking time to fill the body with breath and connect inwardly also helps to relieve fears that may come up about the birth process and the being within. Opening to Grace also will assist in relaxing a woman's mind and allowing her to rest more in her heart.

When practicing yoga — or even while simply finding a quiet moment — the following reflections support Opening to Grace:

> "Open to allow a deeper breath to come in."
> "Feel stronger, brighter from the inside out."
> "Soften to feel the creative pulsations of supreme energy inside."
> "There's a deep inner guidance supporting you — let go of fear."
> "Open to the vast power around you — you are never alone."

Muscular Energy provides strength for a woman in all phases of her pregnancy, particularly as hormones like relaxin take effect, loosening her joints (mainly around the pelvis) creating instability and general discomfort. As a woman's belly grows, the weight of her baby causes her abdominal muscles to stretch far beyond their normal state, losing their ability to help maintain good posture and adding to the lower back 'load.' Engaging Muscular Energy overall will help a woman maintain her strength as well as align her body most optimally. The remembrance to 'hug the muscles' of her physical body also remind a woman to engage the whole process of pregnancy more fully, creating a sense of power in her pregnancy.

The following prenatal reflections support Muscular Energy:

> "Give yourself an unconditional hug by sweetly engaging your muscles."
>
> "Connect to the strength within you."
>
> "Truly commit to your pregnancy."
>
> "Dive into the wisdom of the body."
>
> "Engage the process of creation."
>
> "Feel stable knowing that you are supported."

Inner Spiral reminds a woman that there is always more potential to tap into, whether it is to help relieve physical pain or just expand her perspective about her pregnancy in general. A woman can use Inner Spiral in all trimesters to more precisely open the 'door of the pelvis,' making space to scoop the tailbone and lengthen the lower back (an action of Outer Spiral and a helpful pain reliever). By shifting her weight back, Inner Spiral also gives a woman more freedom to move in a balanced and comfortable way, countering her extra weight that naturally pulls her forward. It is particularly helpful during early stages of labor to help move the baby more into the birth canal and to loosen a woman's inhibitions ultimately supporting the downward flow of energy (*apana vayu*) and the birth of the baby.

Reflections to help a woman connect to the expansive qualities of Inner Spiral are:

> "Grow your image of yourself — see yourself as mother, goddess, woman."
>
> "Make space for your new life."
>
> "Expand your circle, seek community."
>
> "Allow support from others."
>
> "Lavish yourself with attention as your belly grows."

Outer Spiral provides relief and grounds a woman in all phases of her pregnancy, always complementing the freedom created in Inner Spiral. It is key in maintaining length in the lower back, helping to lessen the natural 'sway back' in pregnancy. It is the dynamic pulsation of Inner and Outer Spiral that most often relieves a woman from lower back pain. Outer Spiral also supports a woman during the 'pushing phase' of birth — shortening the distance of the birth canal.

Some Outer Spiral reflections to help a woman feel more grounded include:

"Take time to walk or sit in nature to connect more with the earth."

"Stabilize your inner knowing."

"Organize your home. Be prepared to nest."

"Rehearse your birth plan to feel stable."

"Stay connected to your core beliefs."

Organic Energy supports all the trimesters by reminding a woman to celebrate her pregnancy as sacred. As a woman 'roots' her energy into the earth, she can more fully trust in that which supports her, expanding her perspective of her yoga practice and entire pregnancy. It is particularly helpful during labor if a woman can soften and let 'passive' Organic Energy move through her. This encourages her natural birth hormones (like oxytocin and endorphins) to flow, allowing for an optimal labor and birth.

The following reflections support Organic Energy:

"You are the co-creator of your own reality."

"Fully participate in the currents of Grace."

"Become more fluent in the wisdom of Self."

"Trust in the process of labor and birth."

"Walk through the threshold into motherhood."

PRENATAL ESSENTIALS

NUTRITION

Eating well is essential for both the health of the baby and the mother. A good balanced diet will not only help a woman feel (and look) better throughout her pregnancy, it can help to prevent prematurity and low birth weight in the child. The old saying, "you are what you eat" is never more fitting than during pregnancy — mom needs to remember what she ingests goes right to the baby. She should consider limiting or avoiding all foods and substances that could negatively affect the growing fetus — including caffeine, refined sugar, smoking, and alcohol.

Good nutrition for a pregnant woman begins with eating more protein as well as fruits, nuts, green leafy vegetables, and grains. A pregnant woman should consult with a healthcare practitioner for the desirable amounts and proper intake of folic acid, iron, calcium, fluids, and protein. Pregnant women may also want to drink purified water instead of tap water to avoid lead, excess chlorine, metals, and synthetic hormones. It's also important for a woman to remember to eat small amounts more frequently rather than a few large meals.

Eating well:
- Helps to expand blood volume to meet the increased demands pregnancy makes on the body. Blood bathes and washes over the placenta to help the exchange of oxygen and nutrients.
- Ensures that the uterus and other tissues grow and increase in elasticity and helps the baby grow to his or her full potential.
- May lower the risk of complications like infections, anemia, toxemia, low birth weight, stillbirth, brain damage, and mental retardation.
- Helps to produce good, healthy breast milk.
- Supports a faster recovery for the mother after birth.

PRENATAL YOGA

Prenatal yoga provides the foundation to support and empower a woman throughout all stages of her pregnancy. It builds confidence and trust — infusing a positive attitude that carries a woman through birth and into the threshold of motherhood.

Yoga increases overall strength and flexibility, helping to alleviate many common prenatal ailments such as low back pain, sciatica, fatigue, and nausea. Practicing regularly can help to reduce swelling and inflammation around the joints, promoting circulation of blood and oxygen throughout the body. As the baby grows and there is less space for mom's internal organs, the fluid movements of yoga support both healthy digestion and regularity. Through optimally aligning the physical body, yoga opens the hips, supports the spine, and tones the pelvic floor muscles, better preparing a woman for both labor and physical birth.

Yoga also encourages a woman to trust in her greater connection to the Universe, providing the emotional support to let go of unwarranted (but completely normal) fears and step into the flow of Grace in the most natural and sublime way. Through connecting to the breath, a woman learns to deeply relax and tune in to the natural rhythms inside — reducing anxiety and stress. Yoga empowers a woman to feel deeply connected to her baby during pregnancy.

Group prenatal yoga classes provide a resourceful community of support and often lead to new friendships for mom (and baby). Sharing personal experiences and information can help to quiet anxious feelings and aid in decision-making. Being a part of a yoga studio also offers a perfect haven for a pregnant woman to connect to a larger *kula* (community) of open-hearted people.

Things to remember while practicing yoga:
- Keep the breath smooth and even — avoid any breathing exercises that hold the breath.
- Always create space for the baby — use props when necessary.
- Never push or force a pose — attune to the body, mind, and breath to know when to back off or come out of a pose completely.
- Keep feet at least hip width apart.
- Take as many breaks as needed.
- Strength over flexibility — keep back muscles strong.
- Maintain good alignment using the Universal Principles of Alignment.
- Practice kegels often (see page 34).
- Keep water nearby, rest, take bathroom breaks when needed.
- Do not overheat! It takes the baby 30 minutes longer to cool once mom does (baby is 10-12 degrees warmer than the room).

• Do Savasana on the left side with any necessary props to bring maximum blood flow to the baby.

• Everyday is a new day, check in and listen to how the body feels.

What to avoid in yoga practice:

• Jumping in or out of poses, including Chaturanga.

• Low back twists, anything closing the belly.

• Deep lunges, which can strain the ligaments in the front of the pelvis and destabilize the sacrum due to the hormone relaxin. Focus on strengthening muscles in the legs and around the pelvic floor while stretching.

• Abdominal crunches.

• Overstretching — particularly the belly and the ligaments around the pelvis and the sacrum. Go slowly into backbends and hip openers with increased engagement (once ligaments are overstretched, they can remain that way after pregnancy).

• Arm balances that 'grip' the abdomen or create less space in the belly.

• Forward bends that compress the belly.

• Lying flat on the back after the 4th month — helps avoid the weight of the baby pressing into the inferior vena cava (vein to heart). This may result in dizziness in the mother and loss of blood and oxygen to mother and baby. To be safe, elevate the head and heart with a blanket at least five degrees.

Poses to be cautious of:

• Inversions should not be done with new students to yoga. Experienced practitioners should consider avoiding inversions during weeks 10-13, which is when the placenta is adhering to the uterus. (Legs up the wall provides the same benefits as inversions).

• Backbends can overstretch ligaments and abdominals and destabilize the sacrum.

• Pigeon — this deep hip opener can strain the groins and cause sacral shifts. It can be difficult for beginners to get into and hard on the knees. Experienced practitioners should make sure they are engaging Muscular Energy fully if they wish to continue this pose during pregnancy. Once they are overstretched, ligaments may not return to their pre-pregnancy state.

• Balancing poses that may create instability. Use the wall to avoid falling.

Modifying a non-prenatal yoga class:

The following modifications are useful if prenatal classes are not available or if a pregnant woman wishes to continue taking open classes:

- A pregnant woman should inform the teacher of her pregnancy and any specific conditions/injuries that may be relevant.
- Have two blocks, a strap, a bolster, and/or extra blankets nearby.
- Modify all twists by 'opening up' in the opposite direction (rather than constricting the belly).
- When moving one leg forward from Down Dog to the top of the mat, bring the foot and leg out, up, and around from the side of the hip then back to the center of the mat (avoid crunching the belly).
- Keep the hands elevated on blocks for lunges and both hands inside the bent front leg.
- Bring the knees to the floor for Chaturanga, and place a bolster or blanket under the thighs for Cobra (to give the belly more space). Or skip both of these poses.
- Try to do Prenatal Sun Salutations instead of traditional Sun Salutations (see page 67):
    - Start at the back of the mat with a bolster or blocks in front.
    - Fold into Uttanasana with hands on a bolster or blocks.
    - Walk hands from Uttanasana to Down Dog.
    - Modify Chaturanga with knees on the floor.
    - Do Cobra with a bolster under thighs or skip it and do extra push-ups or a seated shoulder stretch.
    - Walk hands back to feet from Down Dog to Uttanasana.
- Use the wall when needed for all balancing poses, especially for inversions.
- Do not partner up with inexperienced students; a pregnant woman should consider partnering only with the teacher.
- Follow the "what to avoid" list on page 31 regardless of what everyone else is doing. Take Malasana or Virasana and practice kegels if the class is doing poses not suitable for a pregnant woman.
- Read the Prenatal Yoga Quick Reference Page (page 44) before practicing.
- Do Savasana on the left side, using props to increase comfort.
- Don't forget to drink water!

BREATH

The breath is the Divine's manifestation into each of us. It is the very thing that connects us all in life, and yet each of us has our own experience of it. Pregnancy is the only time when two heartbeats (mother and child) share one breath. Through the breath, the mother can consciously communicate her innermost feelings to her baby. The more lovingly a woman brings her awareness to the breath, the more it naturally expands and relaxes into both her and her baby.

Cultivating a yogic breath called '*ujjayi*' is a powerful tool to help a woman calm the mind and relax the body throughout her pregnancy and in the early stages of labor. *Ujjayi* breathing can be done by tightening the glottis muscles in the back of the throat and making a whisper-like sound on both inhalation and exhalation. As active labor progresses, staying attuned to the breath will help a woman remain more deeply in her 'primal zone' — allowing the proper hormones to be released, the cervix to naturally dilate, and stronger contractions to occur that ultimately support delivery. The breath becomes a wonderful companion for a woman to feel less tension mentally and physically and can support her in fully participating (and enjoying!) the birth process.

Pranayama (expanding the breath through various breathing exercises) is a great way for a woman to build concentration, focus the mind, and connect more fully to her baby. The word '*prana*' literally means life force and is the key to all health and wellbeing. *Prana* is also described as the divine Goddess Shakti. Rather than controlling *prana* (the Goddess), we learn to dance with her. The more a woman can connect to the pulsations of Shakti, the more energy, clarity, and peace she will feel during pregnancy, and the more she will experience her labor with greater understanding.

Breathing Exercises

Slow *Ujjayi* Breathing — Expand the breath slowly and evenly, cultivating a rich smooth sound. Begin to put a count to the inhalation. Start with four and increase the count as necessary (when easy). Make sure the beginning and the end of each inhalation is even, rather than drawing in more breath quickly and tapering off at the end. Then, just as deeply and smoothly, exhale the breath for the same count as the inhalation. It is important to remember to not hold the breath.

Alternate Nostril Breathing — Raising the right hand, place the thumb to the right nostril, closing off that side of the nose. Inhale only into the left nostril slowly and evenly. Then closing the left nostril with the ring finger and pinky, exhale only out of the right nostril. Continue to alternate right and left sides in this same way for four to eight rounds and then release the hand and breathe naturally a few breaths. Do not hold or retain the breath.

Sitali **Breath** — This is a sipping breath that is done by breathing through a curled tongue (long sides fold towards each other, creating a tube-like shape) on the inhalation, and then closing the mouth and exhaling through the nostrils. It is especially helpful to do when a woman is hot; the inhalation has a cooling quality when drawn in this way.

Grounding Breath — Take a slow deep inhalation through the nose, then exhale through the mouth making a whispering 'ha' sound. This breath also has a cooling quality and helps to ground a woman's energy at the end of her yoga practice or just simply to relieve stress. Use when needed. Even just three slow breaths can make a difference!

Note: Pregnant women should **NEVER** hold their breath while practicing *pranayama*.

KEGELS

Kegels were originally developed by Dr. Arnold Kegel (kay-gill) to help women with problems controlling urination. They are designed to strengthen and give a woman voluntary control of the pubococygeus muscle (P.C. muscle for short.) Doing kegels helps to maintain and restore lost muscle tone due to childbirth. They are a must! An easy way to locate the P.C. muscle is to stop and start the flow of urine while on the toilet (although this is not a good way to regularly do these exercises). Kegel exercises can be done anywhere and should be done repeatedly and frequently. A pregnant woman should consider trying to do them every time she is waiting for the traffic light to turn green, while waiting for public transportation, watching TV, or checking e-mail — anything she does multiple times a day.

Kegel Exercises

- **Slow Kegels** — tighten the P.C. muscle for a slow count of four. Visualize the muscle slowly rising up like an elevator, from the ground up to each floor. Hold it for four counts at the top floor (without holding the breath) and then release the muscle slowly to the count of four. As the muscle gets stronger, increase the count. Practice for a couple minutes at a time.

- **Quick Kegels** — tighten and relax the P.C. muscle continuously for 30 seconds to one minute. Try doing it while holding yoga postures.

Kegels exercises are also imperative to do AFTER the baby is delivered (vaginally). Many women find their pelvic floor muscles so stretched that they have difficulty laughing hard or sneezing without the escape of some urine. Kegels will strengthen the inner pelvic muscles and may even make sexual intercourse more enjoyable.

SQUATTING

Squatting is considered the birthing position in many cultures. It can increase the pelvic floor by 30% and should be practiced regularly throughout pregnancy to aid in vaginal childbirth. If it is difficult for a woman to get her heels to the ground, she should place a blanket underneath them to stabilize the legs and help get extension in the spine. Squatting is a great place to practice kegels and can be done comfortably leaning against a wall and sitting on a block. In addition, longer squats (at least one minute) with the support of the wall can be great practice for the endurance of a contraction.

Once a woman reaches her third trimester, she should place a block or two underneath her sitting bones while squatting. This is to ensure that the muscles and ligaments in the pelvic floor do not overstretch due to the excess weight from the baby. Place the block in a horizontal position under the sitting bones, and use more than one block if needed. If the baby is breech, a woman should no longer squat after 34 weeks to avoid the baby's buttocks from getting lodged into her pelvis. If a woman has hemorrhoids (which are common during pregnancy) she should avoid squatting as soon as they develop.

MEDITATION AND IMAGERY

It is important for a woman to give herself quiet time everyday to reduce stress and create a deeper connection with herself and her baby. Meditation awakens this inner relationship and opens the heart to experience more joy and trust. Meditation can help a woman explore her deepest hopes and fears about pregnancy and being a parent and support her in visualizing the birth she wants. It also can help her more easily express her feelings to others with love and trust. Regular practice increases positive emotions like love and compassion and helps to dissolve negative emotions and fears. It also strengthens the immune system, calms the nervous system, and increases brain function.

A wonderful way for a woman to honor the powerful time of pregnancy is to create a sacred place in her house (even just a spot) to spend time breathing, visualizing, and meditating daily. She can decorate the area with images that inspire and empower her, and take refuge in this sacred space during labor.

During pregnancy, I recommend sitting in Virasana or Sukhasana using blocks or blankets under the sitting bones. To begin the process of meditation, it may be helpful to use a timer. Start with ten minutes (or less) and then gradually increase the time as it becomes easier to sit longer. Try to use a timer with a soft chime rather than a jarring ring. Put on soothing music to help encourage a greater ability to 'let go.' Expand the breath evenly, allowing the mind to rest on its natural pulsation. Once the mind has been drawn inward and the body feels calm, allow the breath to soften. Let the whole body simply pulsate, visualizing each cell filled with healing energy and light. Continue to visualize this same thing for the baby creating a deep feeling of connection and peace within. Another helpful way for beginners to meditate is by using guided meditation CDs. Some women even like to play them during early stages of labor to help relax.

The following affirmations can be brought into meditation to help ease a woman's fears about childbirth:

- "I feel deeply connected to this miracle of life growing within me."
- "I trust that everything will be exactly the way it is meant to be."
- "I open and surrender to the Divine energy that is guiding the baby and me."

- "With every breath, I feel stronger yet more deeply relaxed."
- "The baby and I are rested and ready."
- "My body knows what to do; I can relax."
- "As the uterus contracts, it's just an amazing 200 lbs of PRESSURE, not pain."
- "The Goddess and I dance together during contractions."

EDUCATION

Spending time researching pregnancy and birth, through online resources, books, and professionals, may be useful for a pregnant woman to understand what is going on within and empower her to trust the pregnancy and birthing process (see the Suggested Reading List on page 78).

Learning about the baby's stages of growth throughout the pregnancy will create a deeper connection between a woman and her baby. It also will help her better understand her own physical changes. Look online for pregnancy sites that offer daily or weekly updates (see the Online Resources section on page 80).

Networking through the yoga community (*kula*) can offer a woman lasting relationships that honor and empower her choices. Exploring childbirth options, as well as vaccination and circumcision options, will allow a woman to feel more confident during critical decision-making.

Research the assistance of a doula to provide physical, emotional, and informational support for women and their partners during labor and birth. The word doula in Greek means 'one who serves a woman' and now has become known as a professional trained in childbirth. The doula's main role is to help women have safe and empowering birthing experiences. Research has shown using a doula decreases the overall cesarean rate, shortens labor, and reduces epidurals and the use of analgesia. Visit dona.org for more information on doulas and locating a doula in your area.

THE THREE TRIMESTERS

FIRST TRIMESTER — (first 12 weeks)

For many women, the first trimester can be an exciting time — particularly if it's the first pregnancy. As the body begins its miraculous reshaping and hormonal levels change, it also can be a bumpy ride! Some women experience extreme nausea throughout the day, while others are fortunate to feel nothing or just a little sick in the morning hours. Eating a few saltine crackers before getting up out of bed (and waiting 20 minutes for them to absorb the stomach acids) can sometimes alleviate this nausea. It is common for women to feel extra tired or hungry — both with good reason considering how much work the body is doing. There are always the lucky ones that feel perfectly fine throughout their entire pregnancy!

The following is a general list of some things to look for in the first trimester:

- Hormone levels increase.
- Mood swings and anxiety.
- Frequent urination (particularly at night as urination helps to eliminate fluid accumulating in the tissues during the day).
- Water retention.
- Feelings of nausea and fatigue.
- Increased appetite.
- Breast size may increase (preparing for breastfeeding).
- Joints between the pelvic bones widen and become more movable around the tenth or eleventh week. Separating bones can pinch the sciatic nerve.
- Constipation.
- Sensitivity to tastes and smells.

SECOND TRIMESTER — (13-26 weeks)

Usually by the second trimester the nausea subsides and energy levels go up (unfortunately not always). Women may find themselves seeking more physical activity and enjoying the company of others. All of the senses in the body heighten and certain smells or tastes are repulsive while others become extraordinary. The second trimester is generally thought of as the 'best' time in pregnancy, enabling travel or pursuing interests that would be difficult once the baby arrives.

The following is a general list of some things to look for in the second trimester:

- Increased energy (compared with the first trimester).
- By the 4th month, the fetus takes up more space.

- By the 5th month, a woman may be able to feel the movements of the fetus (although they actually begin much earlier around 7-8 weeks).
- Waist becomes thicker, womb swells.
- Weight gain.
- Blood volume increases.
- Blood pressure lowers.
- Line from navel to pubic region may darken.
- Increase in salivation.
- Increase in sweat production, which helps eliminate waste.
- Cramps in legs and feet.
- Varicose veins.
- Vivid dreams.
- General fears (baby disabilities, death, parenting concerns, etc…).

THIRD TRIMESTER — (27-38 weeks)

By the third trimester, women are likely to slow down as the weight of the baby makes it more difficult to get around and breathe. Taking naps will help keep energy levels up. Eating smaller meals and more frequently will help alleviate heartburn due to lack of space in the stomach. Balance may become an issue and swelling in the feet, ankles, and hands are all common. Towards the end of the term, the uterus begins to prepare for its big push by contracting in what is known as 'false labor' or Braxton Hicks contractions. Other symptoms in the third trimester include:

- Shortness of breath due to pressure on the lungs from the uterus.
- Diaphragm may be moved as much as an inch.
- Widening of the rib cage to allow for more breath.
- Stomach pushed up, indigestion.
- Difficulty sleeping.
- Walking differently for balance, leaning back to counter weight.
- Back aches (from leaning back), and pelvic joints more separated.
- Possible swelling (edema) in extremities (feet, ankles, hands).
- Uterus contracts and hardens (Braxton Hicks).
- Abdominal muscles separate.
- Fear and excitement about labor and delivery.
- A greater desire to 'nest.'

PRENATAL FACTS

- The length of an average pregnancy is 240-300 days. Doctors generally calculate the due date by going back to the first day of a woman's last menstrual cycle.

- Almost immediately after conception, a woman's hormonal levels increase dramatically. This increase is essential to maintain the right conditions to nourish the baby, help to prepare the uterus for birth, stimulate contractions, and regulate breastfeeding/milk production.

- Progesterone, which is known as the "bonding" hormone, increases up to 100 times in a pregnant woman. It has many roles related to the development of the fetus. Estrogen also increases up to 100 times and helps soften and relax smooth muscle tissue, increasing space in her body for the growing baby and additional demands on her body.

- The placenta produces the hormone relaxin, which softens connective tissue and ligaments, and mobilizes the spinal and pelvic joints. The baby produces the hormone prostaglandin, which thins the cervix and initiates labor.

- A baby begins to move around seven or eight weeks, stretching his/her arms and legs. A mother will begin to feel the movements around the fourth or fifth month.

- A baby recognizes his/her mother's voice by the fourth or fifth month.

- By the end of a pregnancy, the fluids in the body (cells, tissues, and blood) can increase up to 12 pints. The heart's pumping power also has to increase to meet the demands of the blood volume increase (9 pints).

- The length of a contraction is approximately one minute. Contractions move in a wave-like motion from the top of the uterus to the bottom. Strong contractions during active labor generally come every 3-4 minutes and can last as long as ninety seconds.

PREGNANCY CONDITIONS

Here are some common pregnancy conditions and possible ways to alleviate discomfort.

Backaches — maintain good posture using the Universal Principles of Alignment (particularly focusing on Inner and Outer Spiral — see page 23). Try pelvic rocking, thigh stretches, prenatal massage, and visiting a chiropractor specializing in pregnancy.

Breech (at 30-35 weeks) put gentle pressure on baby's head to move. See spinningbabies.com. Try acupuncture, moxibustion (a traditional Chinese medicine technique that involves the burning of mugwort), light and music between the legs. Try communicating with the baby.

Some yoga poses to support flipping the baby include:
- Supported Down Dog with a block under the head or someone holding a strap around the hips and through the inner thighs.
- Quarter Dog: knees on the floor, hips higher than the head and heart.
- Supported backbends with a bolster, blanket, or blocks.
- Inverted L-pose (if comfortable).
- Headstand (if comfortable).

Carpal tunnel syndrome — strengthen the wrists with good Anusara yoga shoulder principles. Elevate the heels of the hands on a blanket roll/towel during practice. Wearing a splint on the wrist at night also may help alleviate night pain.

Colds — nettie pot the sinuses with un-iodized salt. Breathe in steam of chamomile tea. Take buffered Vitamin C, Zinc, and Vitamin B. Consider homeopathic remedies.

Constipation — eat plenty of fruits and vegetables; increase water intake and other fluids, including prune juice.

Dehydration — drink plenty of water. Stay out of the sun. Minimize caffeine.

Dizziness — Sit or lie down to avoid falling. When practicing yoga: do not bring arms over head, come into child's pose, and rest. Try Bach Flower Rescue Remedy.

Edema (swelling) — drink plenty of water. Elevate legs up the wall if swelling is in the feet, ankles, or legs (lift the head above heart after the 4th month). Sleep on the left side. Avoid sitting or standing too long. If sudden or extreme swelling occurs, check with a health care professional to make sure it is not a sign of preeclampsia.

Excessive heat — rest, practice *sitali* breathing (cooling breath by sipping air through the tongue — see page 34), stay well hydrated.

Headache — due to dehydration: drink water, take electrolytes, and rest. From hormones: drink water, rest, massage lavender essential oil on temples.

Heartburn — eat smaller, more frequent meals. Remain upright for an hour after eating; lying down can irritate the problem. Avoid spicy or greasy foods. Consider homeopathic remedies. Practice Virasana/Supta Virasana with props as necessary.

Hemorrhoids — practice legs up the wall (elevate the head and heart after the 4th month). Avoid squatting. Eat more fruits and vegetables, and drink more fluids.

Indigestion — practice Virasana/supported Supta Virasana. Drink mint tea. Avoid greasy and spicy foods. Eat smaller meals.

Insomnia — drink chamomile tea. Avoid eating close to bedtime. Massage head and neck. Try calcium or magnesium supplement. Practice pelvic rocking. Massage lavender essential oil on feet. Go for a walk, meditate, and do yoga during the day.

Leg cramps — flex foot to engage calf muscles (if they cramp while sleeping). Get adequate calcium intake. Dissolve four tablets of Magnesia Phosphorica 6X in a small glass of warm water. Practice seated (wide legged) forward bends like Upavista Konasana.

Nausea — take some form of ginger: either candy or tea. Acupressure: press center point right below the wrist. Eat: have crackers next to the bed, and eat before sitting up. Make sure to have snacks handy when going out. Avoid inversions and Down Dog. Try standing thigh stretches.

Overdue (or due) — massage pressure points: three fingers above inner ankle bone and hand at break between thumb and index finger. Exercise — walking or climbing stairs.

Pelvic pain — regular exercise will help. Rest if painful, or try warm compresses.

Placenta previa — (when the placenta grows in the lowest part of the uterus and covers all or part of the opening to the cervix.) Reduce activities, stay on bedrest, and see a doctor.

Preeclampsia (pregnancy hypertension) — to prevent elevated blood pressure, make sure to eat a well-balanced diet. See a nutritionist specializing in prenatal care.

Restless leg syndrome — (central nervous system disorder which causes an urge to move the legs, associated with an uncomfortable or unpleasant sensation.) Exercise/yoga to stretch and move area. Massage or wrap legs. Place pillow between legs at night. Increase iron intake.

Sciatica — practice Tadasana with a block between the legs using the Universal Principles of Alignment (see section on Inner and Outer Spiral on page 23). Practice standing thigh stretches and Supta Padangustasana.

Stretch marks — eat the proper diet to help skin be healthy. Drink plenty of fluids. Keep the skin hydrated, and massage the belly with shea butter, vitamin E, or almond oil.

Supine hypotensive syndrome — avoid lying flat on the back after the 4th month to prevent possible dizziness and drop of blood pressure caused by weight of uterus, baby, placenta, and amniotic fluids compressing the inferior vena cava. This may also reduce blood to mother's heart and amount of oxygen to baby.

Swelling — practice Virasana, legs up the wall (elevate the head and heart after the 4th month), and wrist and ankle circles. Stay well-hydrated.

Toxemia — (elevated blood pressure, protein in urine, fluid retention, preeclampsia or eclampsia/maternal seizures.) This is a very serious condition that needs medical attention right away.

Varicose veins — practice legs up the wall (elevate the head and heart after the 4th month), exercise the pelvic floor and inner thigh muscles, legs up and down (with resistance like theraband), Virasana. Avoid crossing your legs while sitting. Wear support pantyhose.

PRENATAL YOGA QUICK REFERENCE PAGE

Here are some general prenatal yoga tips and guidelines for all yoginis who have begun the amazing journey into motherhood. First thing to remember is that every pregnancy is different, even for the same woman. It is always best to listen to your body and do only what feels right for you each day. If you are new to yoga, now is not the time for over-achieving. Take it easy, especially when trying new poses. Concentrate more on alignment and breathing deeply.

The first eight weeks... Don't stress if you did something 'not recommended.' Most women don't even know they're pregnant until at least the 5th week! As far as yoga goes, you can continue your regular practice if it feels okay — keeping in mind not to over do it.

8-10 weeks... Now that you know you are pregnant, you'll start feeling the changes in your body. It's time to begin to modify your yoga. Don't over work and get dehydrated! (Your heart rate should not go past 150 bpm.) No excessive twisting or tightening of the abdominals.

If you feel sick, listen to your body and rest more. Let go of the idea that you have to have the perfect body when you're pregnant and eat. It is fine to continue your regular yoga practice (being mindful of the precautions listed on pages 31–32 and paying close attention to how you are feeling), but it is a good time to start learning how to modify your poses.

10-13 weeks... This is a time when you want to lay low and make sure everything sticks. Take it really easy, relax more, and don't push yourself in your yoga practice. No inversions for this period, especially anything that may be jarring, like kicking up into handstands.

13 weeks... After this time, no deep twists that tighten the belly. You may have noticed that it's growing. Take care in backbends that overstretch the belly. You may have to ease up on these for a while until they feel better.

2nd trimester... If you weren't feeling so great during your first trimester, rejoice, relief is in sight. The nausea should subside, and you may notice that you have more energy now. If you love inversions, now is the time to put them back in. Headstands and handstands are safe if they feel okay — but always use a wall or ask the teacher for support (your center of gravity and ability to balance may shift day-to-day). If they are new for you, wait until after your baby arrives to start. Your yoga practice should consist mainly of standing poses, squats, shoulder and hip openers and strengtheners, gentle forward bends, breathing exercises, and kegels. Try to avoid tightening your belly in all poses. Keep your knees on the floor in Chaturanga and do nothing directly on your belly — your baby likes lots of space. And remember, drink water.

By the end of the fourth month, because of your growing uterus, lying flat on your back could put excessive weight on major blood vessels cutting off oxygen to you and your baby. This does not happen for everyone — and you will feel dizzy before the baby is in any danger. But to be safe, place a blanket under your upper back at a five degree incline to keep your head above your heart. The most optimal resting position is on your left side since this brings maximum blood flow to baby...that means Savasana on your left.

3rd trimester... You're getting pretty good at knowing what you can and can't do by now. Continue to modify poses using props, and avoid doing anything that closes the front of your body and overstretches your ligaments. Keep your legs wide apart for seated poses, and don't push too far. Some days you'll have energy for your practice and other days you won't. Remember to do your kegel exercises regardless. Try doing restorative poses that calm the mind and help you connect to your baby. This is such a magical time. Make sure you slow down enough to enjoy this miracle of life within you. If you haven't been to prenatal classes yet, now is the time. It's a wonderful way to connect with other women and make lasting new friendships for you and your baby.

ESSENTIAL OILS FOR PREGNANCY

Aromatherapy uses pure essential plant oils to enhance and restore health by stimulating the body's own natural healing process. There are different qualities or 'grades' of essential oils, and it is very important that a pregnant woman use the highest quality 'therapeutic' grade when trying out any oil. This section includes a list of essential oils to avoid and a list of those that are safe for pregnant women to use during specific times of their pregnancy and childbirth. I have noted whether they are 'safe throughout' (s.t.) or to be used only after a certain number of weeks. Essential oils should always be diluted in carrier oils during pregnancy (vegetable oils, sweet almond oil, grape seed oil, jojoba oil, etc…) for topical treatments and massage (two drops of essential oil for every teaspoon of carrier oil).

A good introduction for using essential oils in pregnancy is for a woman to choose an appealing scent and place one drop on a tissue to inhale. If the smell is appealing, she can place the tissue inside her bra and enjoy it the rest of the day. Other options include: adding essential oils to a bath (dilute three to seven drops mixed with a carrier oil before putting into bath), using a device to diffuse oils into a room (ceramic burner, electric diffuser, or vaporizer), and adding four drops to lukewarm water to soak feet, etc. My favorite first choice for a pregnant woman to try is lavender oil, which has many wonderful therapeutic qualities and is safe to use throughout pregnancy.

Please note: Since it would be highly unethical to test on pregnant women, this list of essential oils is based on knowledge of the general properties of each essential oil. It is best to avoid essential oils that are known to thin the blood or cause cramping or contractions. In general, a pregnant woman should err on the side of caution, particularly during the first trimester and consult with her doctor, midwife, or a practitioner trained in the application of essential oils during pregnancy.

The following two companies have superb integrity and high quality therapeutic grade oils:
- Oshadhi: oshadhiusa.com
- Swiss Aromatics: originalswissaromatics.com.

ESSENTIAL OILS TO AVOID DURING PREGNANCY

Basil	Lemongrass
Camphor	Myrrh
Cedarwood	Parsley
Cinnamon	Pennyroyal
Clove	Sage
Fennel	Sweet marjoram
Hyssop	Tansy
Juniper	Thyme

ESSENTIAL OILS TO BE USED WITH CAUTION DURING PREGNANCY

Chamomile, Roman (safe after 16 weeks)

Clary Sage (only late pregnancy)

Cypress (safe after 16 weeks)

Geranium (safe after 16 weeks)

Jasmine (safe after 16 weeks)

Peppermint (safe after 16 weeks)

Rose (safe after 16 weeks)

Rosemary (late pregnancy only, avoid if high blood pressure)

ESSENTIAL OILS SAFE TO USE DURING PREGNANCY

Bergamot	Orange
Frankincense	Patchouli
Grapefruit	Rosewood
Lavender	Sandalwood
Lemon	Tangerine
Mandarin	Tea Tree
Neroli	Ylang Ylang

Note – bergamot, lemon, mandarin, and orange essential oils are phototoxic (can cause skin irritation) and should not be used while in direct sunlight.

COMMON PREGNANCY CONDITIONS SUPPORTED BY ESSENTIAL OILS

It is important for a pregnant woman to seek the council of a qualified aromatherapist before administering essential oils on her own to alleviate ailments.

Backache — roman chamomile (after 16 wks), rosemary (late pregnancy), lavender (s.t.).

Depression and anxiety — bergamot (s.t.), roman chamomile (after 16 wks), frankincense (s.t.), geranium (after 16 wks), neroli (s.t.), ylang-ylang (s.t.), rose (after 16 wks).

Edema (swelling) — geranium (after 16 wks), grapefruit (s.t.).

Feeling lethargic — orange (s.t.), peppermint (after 16 wks).

Headaches — lavender (s.t.), peppermint (after 16 wks).

Healing damaged tissue — tea tree (s.t.), lavender (s.t.).

Hormonal equilibrium — geranium (after 16 wks), jasmine (good for after childbirth), rose (good for after childbirth).

Indigestion— lavender (s.t.).

Immune system booster — lemon (s.t.), lavender (s.t.).

Induce labor/strengthen contractions — clary sage (only late pregnancy- stimulates and tones uterus).

Inflamed skin — lavender (s.t.).

Insomnia — lavender (s.t.).

Muscle spasm — roman chamomile (after 16 wks).

Nausea — lavender (s.t.), peppermint (after 16 wks).

Poor circulation — geranium (after 16 wks), lemon (s.t.).

Postpartum depression — vetiver, lemon, cedarwood, sandlewood, St. John's wort.

Relaxing, calming, optimism — jasmine (after 16 wks), roman chamomile (after 16 wks), mandarin (s.t.), rose (after 16 wks), sandalwood (s.t.).

Settles digestive tract — mandarin (s.t.), orange (s.t.), peppermint (after 16 wks), lavender (s.t.).

Settles nervous system — mandarin (s.t.), neroli (s.t.), rose (after 16 wks).

Stress — lavender (s.t.), frankincense (s.t.), geranium (after 16 wks).

Stretch marks — neroli (s.t.).

Varicose veins/hemorrhoids — cypress (after 16 weeks).

PERINEAL MASSAGE USING CARRIER OIL

During the last six weeks of a woman's pregnancy, she may want to try massaging her perineum for five or six minutes a day to prevent tearing or the need for an episiotomy during delivery.

To begin, she can take a warm bath or shower to help relax the tissues. Using a nut-based carrier oil such as almond oil, she can begin by simply massaging her perineum and lower vaginal wall. After a couple of minutes, she should begin to use both of her thumbs inside the vagina and press down towards her rectum. Maintaining steady pressure, she should move her thumbs in a "U" type movement and then hold for 30-60 seconds, then release. If she feels a slight burning or tingling sensation, she can try relaxing her pelvic floor muscles. This is what she must do when the baby's head begins to crown in birth. At first this tissue will feel tight, but with time it will stretch and relax. The exercise should not be painful, and she can seek her care provider's help if she has difficulty or questions.

PREPARING FOR LABOR AND BIRTH WITH YOGA

The extraordinary journey of pregnancy culminates in the process of giving birth. It is likely to be among the most powerful and monumental experiences for both the mother and child. Yoga supports this sacred passage by preparing a woman both physically and emotionally — offering her resources for before, during labor, and even after the baby arrives.

During the last six weeks or so of pregnancy, a woman will experience many different sensations as her body innately prepares for birth. On a physical level, the ligaments in her pelvis are moving towards maximum softness to allow her pelvic and sacroiliac joints to expand. The uterus will begin contracting (Braxton Hicks), which may feel like a powerful tightening or hardening of the abdomen. Usually the baby's head begins to descend into the pelvis during the last four weeks (lightening), potentially increasing contractions. Once she notices a 'dropping' of the baby, she may feel less pressure on her diaphragm making it easier to breathe — but possibly more pressure on her bladder resulting in more frequent urination. (Note: 'lightening' prior to labor is more obvious with first time births because the uterine muscles are tighter and babies are under more downward pressure.)

By utilizing the breath, mantra (affirmations), specific yoga postures, and meditation, a woman can often alleviate discomfort in her lower back and pelvis and even maximize space in the birth canal for the baby's entrance into the world. These practices also help release stiffness and tension in her muscles, keeping her body softer and more capable of relaxing when needed. It is essential for a woman's pelvic floor to relax during childbirth to avoid unwanted tears or an episiotomy — a surgical incision through the perineum made to enlarge the vagina and assist childbirth.

BREATHING EXERCISES FOR LABOR

It is best for a woman to practice awareness of the breath throughout her pregnancy (see grounding breath on page 34). When she begins the first stage of labor she can return to the connection and familiarity of the breath to move her through her contractions. As the contractions build in strength, she should focus on her exhalation, relax as much as possible, and naturally let the inhalation begin. Repeat this cycle through the wave of each contraction until it ebbs.

There is no 'right' way to breathe — it is more important that a woman is comfortable with what she is doing. As the labor progresses into the second stage (bearing down), this is essential. Some women are taught to take a huge breath, hold it, and push, while others may be encouraged to relax into the contraction and surrender. A safe answer is to encourage a woman to keep breathing deeply (this supplies maximum oxygen for herself and her baby), concentrate on opening and relaxing on her exhale, and center her awareness on releasing all tension in her pelvic floor to aid in the arrival of her baby. Studies have shown that releasing the mouth and jaw may correspond to a release in the pelvic floor.

MANTRAS (AFFIRMATIONS) FOR LABOR

Sound plays an important role in enabling a woman to let go. As the labor progresses, she will find it very difficult to tolerate outside sounds or disturbances. Many women turn inward, finding a comfortable place to open to her deep primal urge to sound. Having a 'mantra,' which is simply a sound, syllable, or group of words that she can repeat over and over again, will help her move more deeply into a trance-like state. It also helps her relax her lips and mouth, which may have a similar effect on loosening her cervix.

Some possible mantras she can repeat are:
- 'Om.'
- 'Aaaaaaah, Uuuuuu, Mmmm' (Aum translates to Om).
- 'So hum' (I am that).

Some possible affirmations she can repeat are:
- 'Opening and surrendering.'
- 'Inhale/exhale.'
- 'Each contraction brings me closer to meeting my baby.'
- 'Wow, 200 lbs of pressure, not pain.'

- 'All is well.'
- 'With grace and ease.'
- 'I am (fill in the blank)' — i.e strong, ready, etc.
- 'Oh yes.'

YOGA POSTURES FOR LABOR

A woman will naturally move in a variety of positions during labor to help alleviate discomfort and relax her body. It is helpful for her to get to know the following yoga postures beforehand so she can support these natural instincts during labor.

Standing Tadasana: works with gravity to assist the baby moving downward, helps thin the cervix.

Modified Tadasana: leaning forward with her arms around a partner's neck, she can 'hang' on her exhalation and have her partner massage her back.

Supported Tadasana: put a strap around the top of a door and holding the strap with both hands, let her body 'hang' on contractions with her exhalations and mantra.

Supported Balasana (child's pose): knees wide, torso resting over a chair or pillows. This is a good position to have a partner massage her back.

Squatting: helps put pressure on the cervix to open and shortens the distance of the birth canal. This position is best to use as labor progresses as it makes contractions more intense.

Modified squatting: sitting on the edge of a chair with her knees wide, leaning forward slightly.

Partner squatting: have a partner stand behind with his/her forearms under her armpits, allowing her to bend her knees half way and let go on contractions.

Supported deep squat: have a partner support her from behind in a squat or low chair.

All fours/pelvic rocking: relieves lower back pain by taking the weight of baby away from her spine. Also allows for less pressure on her tailbone.

Supported all fours: using the support of a chair or pillow for elbows, resting her weight forward.

Supported Savasana (on left side): good position for resting or sleeping, this helps her perineum relax to prevent tearing. This is the preferred position as opposed to lying on her back, which may slow down labor.

Through yoga and meditation, a woman also learns to surrender more and more into her deeper states of consciousness (connectedness), tapping into her most instinctive and primal self (and getting ready to invoke the Goddess Kali when needed). This expansion of awareness, which is natural to feel at the end of pregnancy, will support her immensely if she can flow with it, bringing her more ease and assurance that she is ready, regardless of how her labor progresses.

It is completely normal to feel anxiety and fear wondering about the unknowns of labor. However, the more a woman can face her darkest emotions during pregnancy and open up to the intensity of birth during labor, the more she will be able to access her body's intuitive gifts and return back to her excitement that the baby is coming. If anything, she must learn to 'get out of her own way' and let the inherent wisdom of the body do its job!

It's important for a woman to know that hormones such as oxytocin and endorphins play a significant role in assisting her labor and birth while the hormone adrenaline can actually slow down the process — particularly during the first stage of labor. Oxytocin is a potent stimulator of contractions, which helps to dilate the cervix, move the baby down and out of her body, give birth to her placenta, and limit bleeding. During labor and birth, the pressure of the baby against the cervix and then against tissues in the pelvic floor stimulates oxytocin and contractions. Endorphins are calming and pain-relieving hormones that produce an altered state of consciousness that helps a woman flow with the process, even when it is long and arduous. High endorphin levels can help her feel more euphoric and uninhibited rather than frightened and in pain.

A woman can promote a healthy production of both oxytocin and endorphins during labor and birth by:
- Staying calm, comfortable, and confident.
- Avoiding unwelcome disturbances and people.
- Remaining more upright to use gravity to apply pressure from the baby on the pelvic floor (releasing oxytocin).
- Stimulating her nipples (releasing oxytocin).
- Delaying or avoiding epidural or other prescriptive pain relief.

Adrenaline is the "fight or flight" hormone that humans produce to help ensure survival. A woman who feels threatened during labor (for example by fear or severe pain) may produce high levels of adrenaline. Adrenaline can slow labor or stop it altogether, particularly in the first stage. Earlier in human evolution, this disruption helped birthing women move to a place of greater safety. During the second stage of labor when the expulsive reflex begins, adrenaline may be produced to help a mother gather strength to aid the birth of her baby.

Some ways to keep adrenaline down during labor are:
- Staying calm, comfortable, and relaxed.
- Being informed and prepared.
- Trusting her caregivers and her capabilities.
- Keeping her environment peaceful and private, and avoiding disruption.
- Being comforted with positive words and other support.
- Avoiding intrusive, painful, or disruptive procedures.

While every labor develops its own unique rhythm or pattern and waves of contractions slowly increase in frequency, the process can be distinctly divided into three stages. The first stage of labor can be compared to running a marathon, at times feeling like it's too much and then getting a second wind. The cervix is softening (latent phase) and then fully dilates (active phase). The last phase is called transition, which varies from seconds to hours and is the time when labor begins its 'transition' to the second stage — the expulsive reflex to bear down until the baby is born. The third stage of labor is the joyful union of mother holding child, the birthing of the placenta, and her body's recovery from birth.

Immediately after giving birth, a woman will still experience some aches and pains as her body begins the miraculous journey back to normal. This varies from several days to several weeks depending on whether she had a vaginal birth or a c-section — (a surgical incision made in the abdomen and uterus to deliver the baby). She can continue to practice deep breathing through any cramps and use positive affirmations to stay relaxed and calm. Yoga postures should be avoided until she has stopped bleeding and has been given the okay from her doctor or midwife (see Once the Baby Arrives on page 56).

EMBRACING BIRTH OUTCOME

As much as a woman can plan for her baby's birth, there are no guarantees as to what the outcome will be. This is true whether it is a woman's first delivery or subsequent childbirth experience. The practice of yoga encourages a woman to let go of her expectations around the 'ideal' birth and learn to embrace her journey regardless of how it unfolds. For example, a woman may experience mixed emotions upon learning that she unexpectedly needs a cesarean or if she had planned on giving birth naturally and instead decides she would like pain relief (such as an epidural). In whatever way her labor and delivery unfold, prenatal yoga can provide valuable support.

Using the first principle of Anusara yoga, 'Opening to Grace,' she can use her breath to soften and remember that every experience is an opportunity to connect in deeper ways to herself and the greater, diverse Whole. Rather than seeing her outcome as imperfect, she may choose to celebrate her experience as 'perfect' for herself and equally Divine. Ultimately, regardless of how her baby enters the world, she can step into the threshold of motherhood with Grace.

ONCE THE BABY ARRIVES

Just when a woman thought the marathon was over, welcome to the 4th trimester! Life with baby in arms is certainly more joyous than labor and delivery, but that doesn't mean the first few months postpartum is not seriously challenging as well. Hormonal shifts, which happen immediately and continue the first couple of weeks, can create emotional swings and physical discomfort. Some common things a woman might experience postpartum are:

- Night sweats — as excess water is released from the body.
- Sore breasts — as milk production increases.
- Leaky breasts — if a woman chooses to nurse.
- Hair loss — which usually subsides after 6 months.
- Vaginal soreness — try soaking in sitz baths (a plastic bowl that fits over the toilet seat) and applying frozen pads soaked in healing herbs (only for vaginal births, not c-section).
- Vaginal discharge — blood flow like menstruation (lochia), which should decrease each day.
- Contractions — first few days after birth, similar to menstrual cramps, may increase during nursing.
- Skin changes — blood vessels in face may have increased during the pushing phase (these should gradually fade).
- Hemorrhoids — try soaking in sitz baths (see above) and applying cool compresses.
- Lack of sleep — due to baby's feeding schedule. Sleep when the baby sleeps.
- Leaky bladder — when sneezing or laughing. Do kegels (see page 34).
- 'Baby blues' — onset may occur during the first couple of weeks.
  Note: Some new mothers still experiencing the 'blues' beyond the second week may be one of the 10-20% of women who develop postpartum depression, a serious condition which may require medical attention.

I advise new mothers to do their best to stay home the first six weeks after delivery (offered to me by Gurmukh Khalsa and the Sikh community), which helps the body recover strength and avoid relapsing later in the year. It also allows for essential bonding time between mother and baby as they establish their new rhythm together (which is generally feeding, sleeping, and pooping!). While not all women have that luxury to spend six weeks nesting (especially if it's not their first baby), it is important for new moms to remember to take extra care and not try to be 'super mom'. If a woman doesn't have sufficient help from family members, there are postpartum doulas available to help prepare nourishing meals, clean, tend to baby while mommy sleeps, and do laundry. New mothers having problems or new to nursing can contact La Leche League (llli.org), which offers incredible support and encouragement.

If a woman was able to stay in good shape during her pregnancy and had a healthy vaginal delivery, she can begin light exercise (walking, gentle yoga) within a couple weeks of her delivery. For a c-section, she should wait six to eight weeks to exercise, except light walking which is actually beneficial after a couple of weeks. Most doctors advise waiting until after the six week check-up before resuming a normal exercise routine. Regardless of when a woman decides to start, she needs to remember to go slowly. Her joints and ligaments will still be loose for about three to five months, so she should keep any exercise low-impact and focus on toning and stretching. Also, a woman's abdominal muscles separate during pregnancy and take about four to eight weeks for the gap to close (although usually not fully). If she begins abdominal crunches before the gap is three finger widths or less, she may risk injury. (A way to check the abdominals is to lie flat on the back with the knees bent. On an exhale, lift the head and shoulders, reaching one arm towards the knees to tighten the muscles. Place fingers right above the belly button and see how wide the space is from the center out.)

A nice way for a woman to begin postnatal yoga at home is to first try a few poses she was doing while she was pregnant. Starting with simple breathing and warm-up poses such as cat/cow, she can ease her way into a few different categories of poses. This will give her an awareness of where her body is regarding strength, etc. Then she can begin to add poses that specifically build strength (in the legs, back, abdominals, arms) using the Universal Principles of Alignment (i.e. Down Dog, Plank, Chaturanga, Cobra) as well as those she had to avoid during pregnancy (twists, deep backbends, etc.). When she is ready to venture to class, postnatal or mommy and me classes are a great first option and can be reassuring. If there are no specialty classes available, she should try a beginner yoga class first and let the instructor know she's a new mom.

Most importantly, a woman should be kind to herself regarding her physical appearance and weight. With all the enormous changes taking place during her '4th trimester,' including lack of sleep and a brand new life with little one, there is everything to be proud of and celebrate. Soon enough things fall into place and new routines allow for more personal time. Some of the most powerful moments of a woman's life are during the sweet connections made in the quiet hours when she and baby are communing with the moon.

YOGA SEQUENCES

The following yoga sequences are meant to support the different levels of prenatal yoga practitioners, ranging from beginner to intermediate. Also included are specific sequences for nausea, restoratives, and infertility. It is important for a woman to take extra care not to push herself beyond her current level of yoga experience while she is pregnant to avoid strain or possible injury to herself and her growing baby. For all women, I recommend focusing on the breath and proper alignment (see the section on the Universal Principles of Alignment on page 22), gently opening the body, and keeping up strength. Working with an experienced yoga teacher is always advised, especially for beginners.

Warm Up/Sun Salutations

This routine can be done as a warm-up for a longer practice or simply as a sweet way to 'salute the sun' each new day.

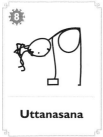

Sukhasana

On blanket for opening meditation.

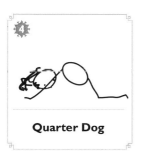

All Fours

Root hands, strengthen arms, soften heart.

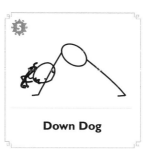

Cat/Cow Pelvic Tilts

5x. Link breath with movement; don't over arch lower back.

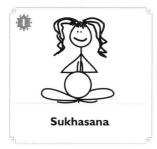

Quarter Dog

Knees on floor, arms angled back, arm bones lift.

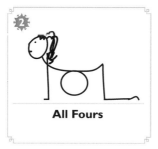

Down Dog

Wide legs, walk feet out.

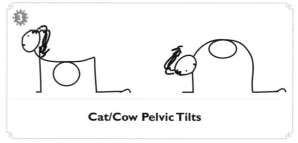

All Fours Variations

Balancing opposite arm/leg.

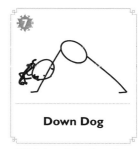

Down Dog

Walk hands back to feet for Uttanasana (standing forward fold).

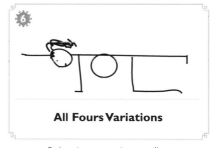

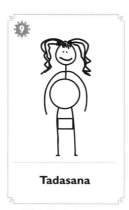

Uttanasana

With hands elevated on blocks if needed, feet wide.

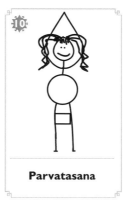

Tadasana

With block between inner thighs.

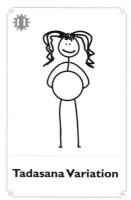

Parvatasana

Arms overhead.

Tadasana Variation

Bound hands/shoulder stretch.

...continued on next page

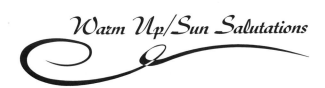

Warm Up/Sun Salutations

...continued from page 59

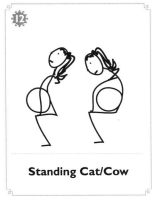

Standing Cat/Cow

Pelvic tilts.

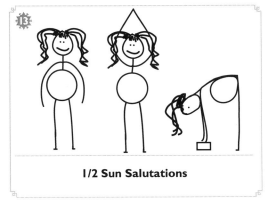

1/2 Sun Salutations

3x. Hands on blocks if needed.

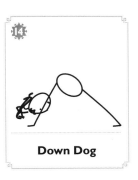

Down Dog

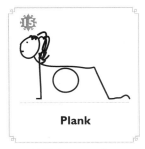

Plank

With knees on floor behind hips.

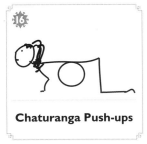

Chaturanga Push-ups

3x. Knees on floor.

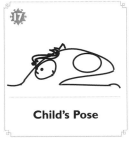

Child's Pose

Knees wide, toes together, arms forward.

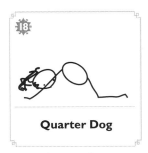

Quarter Dog

Knees on floor.

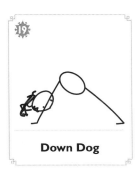

Down Dog

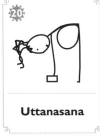

Uttanasana

With hands elevated on blocks if needed, feet wide.

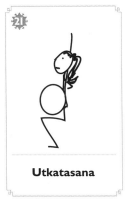

Utkatasana

To modify: either forearms to thighs, arms straight forward, final stage arms up.

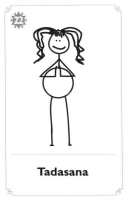

Tadasana

End with 5 deep breaths.

Beginner Sequence

This beginner sequence is safe to do regularly — supporting strength, flexibility, and balance. Note: new students should still seek a teacher to ensure proper alignment.

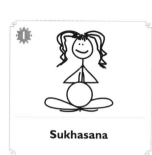

Sukhasana

On blanket for opening meditation.

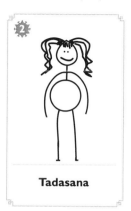

Tadasana

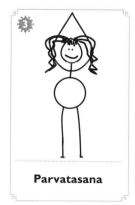

Parvatasana

Arms overhead.

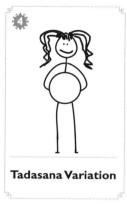

Tadasana Variation

Bound hands/shoulder stretch.

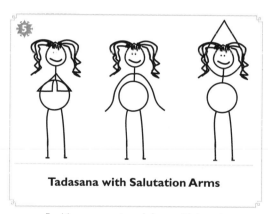

Tadasana with Salutation Arms

5x. Move arms up and down with breath.

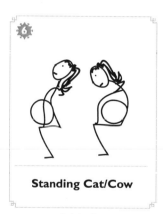

Standing Cat/Cow

Pelvic tilts.

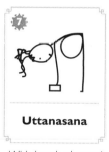

Uttanasana

With hands elevated on blocks if needed, feet wide.

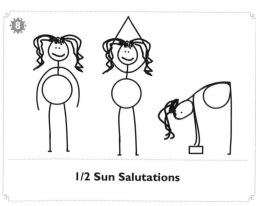

1/2 Sun Salutations

3x. Walk arms forward to all fours.

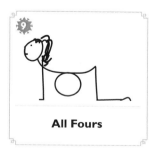

All Fours

Root hands, strengthen arms, soften heart.

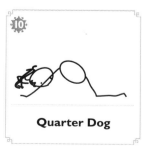

Quarter Dog

Knees on floor, arms angled back, arm bones lift.

...continued on next page

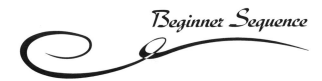

...continued from page 61

Beginner Sequence

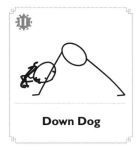

Down Dog

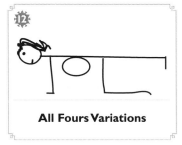

All Fours Variations

Balancing opposite arm/leg.

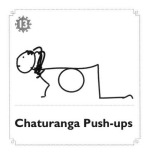

Chaturanga Push-ups

3x. Knees on floor.

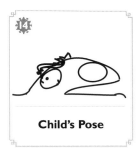

Child's Pose

Knees wide, toes together, arms forward.

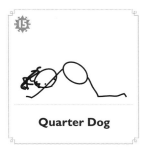

Quarter Dog

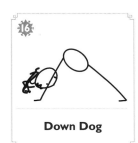

Down Dog

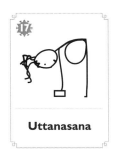

Uttanasana

Bend knees, hands on thighs to stand.

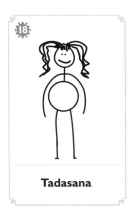

Tadasana

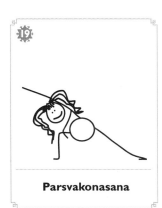

Parsvakonasana

Forearm to thigh or hand to block. Both sides.

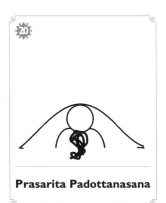

Prasarita Padottanasana

With block under hands if needed. Fold down the middle.

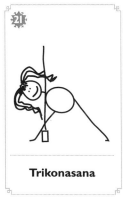

Trikonasana

With block if needed. Both sides.

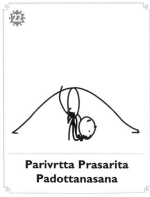

Parivrtta Prasarita Padottanasana

With gentle open-belly twist.

...continued on next page

...continued from page 62

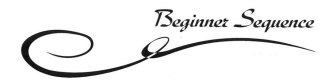

Beginner Sequence

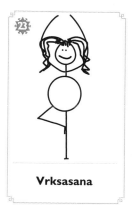

Vrksasana

With wall behind back.

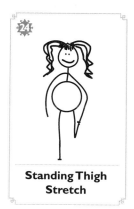

Standing Thigh Stretch

Hold wall if needed, breathe into back body.

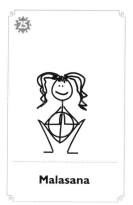

Malasana

At wall, practice kegels, use block under sitting bones if necessary.

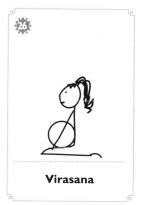

Virasana

Use block or blanket if needed.

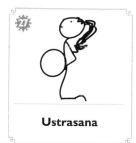

Ustrasana

With slight upper backbend, keep hands on hips.

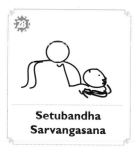

Setubandha Sarvangasana

Gentle lift of hips if comfortable. 3x. Rest on left side in between.

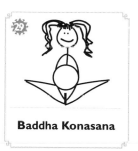

Baddha Konasana

Feet apart to fold forward.

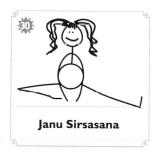

Janu Sirsasana

Fold between the legs.

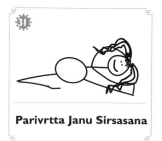

Parivrtta Janu Sirsasana

Place the top hand behind the base of the skull and the bottom hand on the floor.

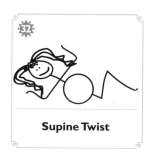

Supine Twist

Knees bent away from belly.

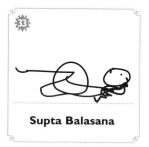

Supta Balasana

Lift head above heart after 4th month.

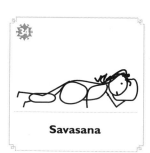

Savasana

With props on left side and between legs.

Wall Sequence (Mixed Level)

The wall is one of the most useful prenatal 'props' — it ensures stability and increases one's ability to engage and open the body. This sequence can be modified according to the level of the practitioner, and poses can be eliminated to shorten the length of the sequence.

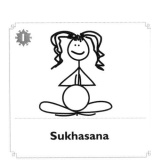

Sukhasana

On blanket for opening meditation.

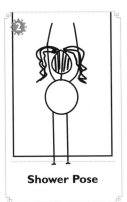

Shower Pose

Standing facing the wall (2 feet away), arms overhead, hands at wall.

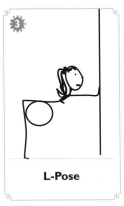

L-Pose

Torso parallel to floor, hips over heels.

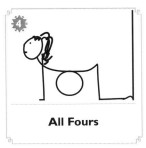

All Fours

Facing away from wall. Root hands, strengthen arms, soften heart.

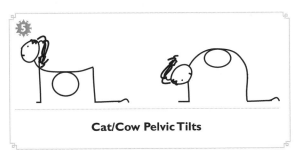

Cat/Cow Pelvic Tilts

5x. Link breath with movement.

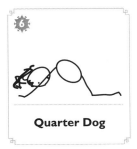

Quarter Dog

Knees on floor, arms angled back, arm bones lift.

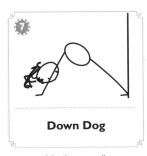

Down Dog

Heels up wall.

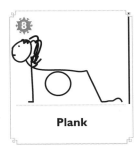

Plank

With knees on floor behind hips.

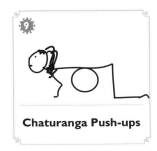

Chaturanga Push-ups

3x. Knees on floor.

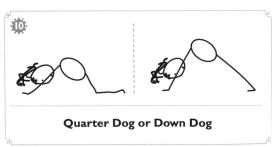

Quarter Dog or Down Dog

Then walk hands back to feet.

...continued on next page

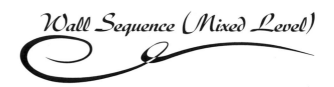

Wall Sequence (Mixed Level)

...continued from page 64

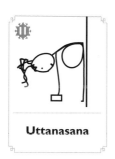

Uttanasana

With hands elevated on blocks if needed. Thighs back towards wall.

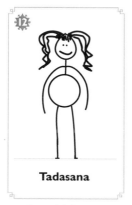

Tadasana

Step slightly away from wall.

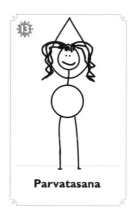

Parvatasana

Arms overhead, lift heels (use wall for balance).

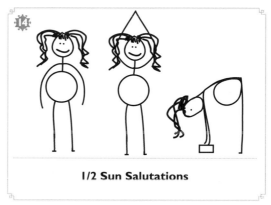

1/2 Sun Salutations

3x. Hands on blocks if needed.

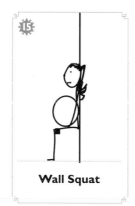

Wall Squat

1 minute. 2x. Lean against wall with block between legs.

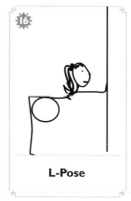

L-Pose

From L-pose, move left foot to wall for standing pose.

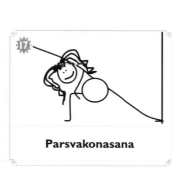

Parsvakonasana

Forearm to thigh or hand to block (back foot pressing against wall).

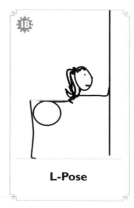

L-Pose

L-pose in between right and left side.

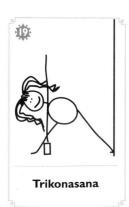

Trikonasana

Use block if needed (back foot pressing against wall).

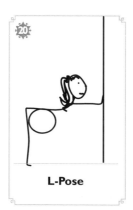

L-Pose

L-pose in between right and left side.

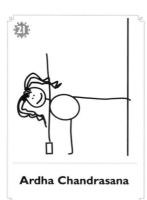

Ardha Chandrasana

With foot on wall or leaning against wall. Use block if needed.

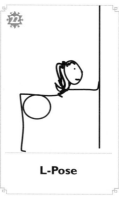

L-Pose

L-pose in between right and left side.

...continued on next page

Wall Sequence (Mixed Level)

...continued from page 65

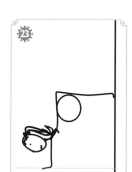

Inverted L-pose

(1/2 handstands) if comfortable.

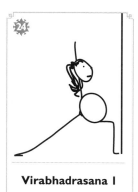

Virabhadrasana I

Facing wall with back heel up – straighten and bend front leg with breath.

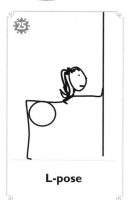

L-pose

Torso parallel to floor, hips over heels.

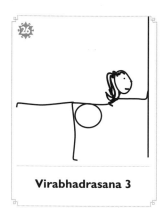

Virabhadrasana 3

With hands at wall, leg lower than hip.

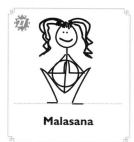

Malasana

At wall – practice kegels.

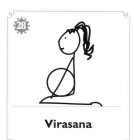

Virasana

Then with slight upper backbend (or supta with block behind back, first trimester only).

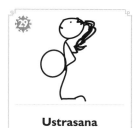

Ustrasana

With slight upper backbend or hands to heels (if comfortable).

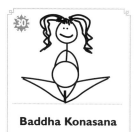

Baddha Konasana

Feet apart to fold forward.

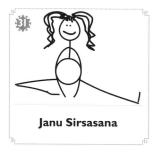

Janu Sirsasana

Fold between legs.

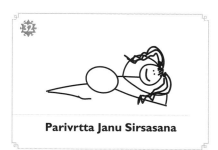

Parivrtta Janu Sirsasana

Place the top hand behind the base of the skull and the bottom hand on the floor.

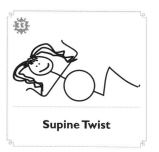

Supine Twist

Knees bent away from belly.

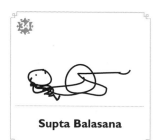

Supta Balasana

Lift head above heart after 4th month.

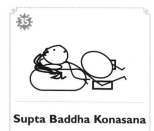

Supta Baddha Konasana

With blocks under knees and bolster under torso.

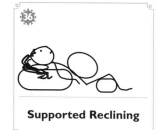

Supported Reclining

With bolster under torso and knees.

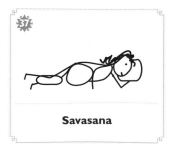

Savasana

With props on left side and between legs.

Intermediate Sequence

This practice is for experienced yoginis comfortable in these poses before getting pregnant. It is advisable to work slowly to decide each day whether to modify or leave out poses.

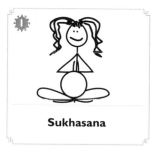

Sukhasana

On blanket for opening meditation.

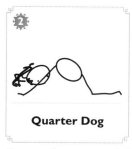

Quarter Dog

Knees on floor, arms angled back, arm bones lift.

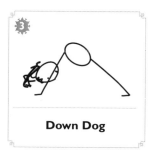

Down Dog

Wide legs, walk feet out. Then, walk hands back to feet.

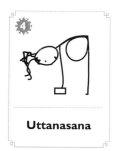

Uttanasana

With hands elevated on blocks if needed.

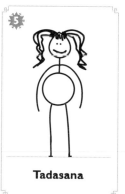

Tadasana

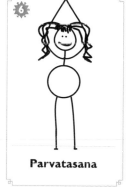

Parvatasana

Arms overhead, then arms clasped behind back.

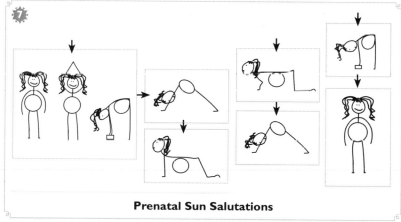

Prenatal Sun Salutations

3x. Walk forward into Down Dog, Plank with knees on floor, Chaturanga, Cobra (if it feels ok), Down Dog, walk hands to feet for Uttanasana, Tadasana.

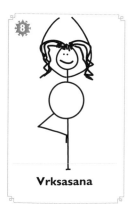

Vrksasana

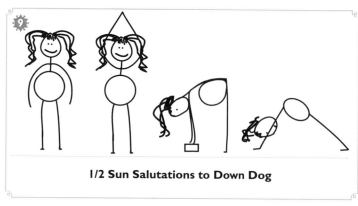

1/2 Sun Salutations to Down Dog

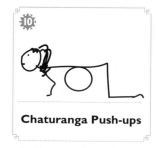

Chaturanga Push-ups

3x. Knees on floor. Lift heels of hands if possible.

...continued on next page

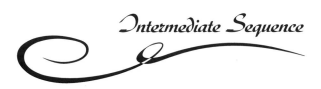

Intermediate Sequence

...continued from page 67

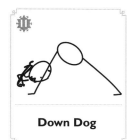

Down Dog

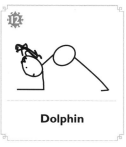

Dolphin

Forearms to floor. Then Down Dog, walk hands to feet.

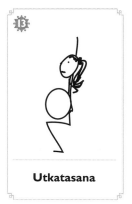

Utkatasana

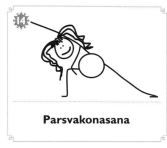

Parsvakonasana

Forearm to thigh or hand to block. Both sides.

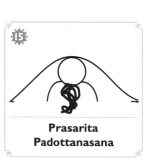

Prasarita Padottanasana

Fold down the middle.

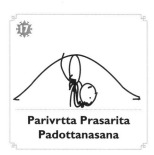

Trikonasana

With block if needed. Both sides.

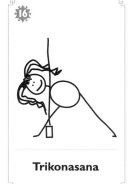

Parivrtta Prasarita Padottanasana

With gentle open-belly twist.

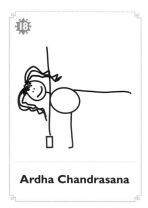

Ardha Chandrasana

With foot on wall or leaning against wall. Use block if needed.

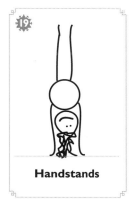

Handstands

Or 1/2 handstands at wall (if comfortable).

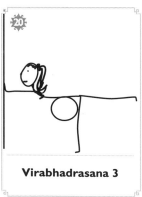

Virabhadrasana 3

Hands at wall, then let go.

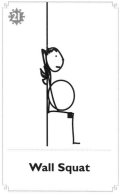

Wall Squat

1 minute. 2x. Lean against wall with block between legs.

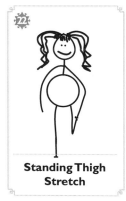

Standing Thigh Stretch

Hold wall if needed, breathe into back body.

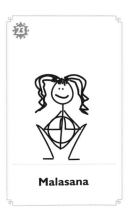

Malasana

Practice kegels.

...continued on next page

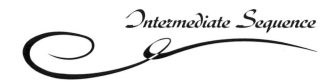
Intermediate Sequence

...continued from page 68

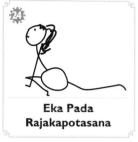

Eka Pada Rajakapotasana

Pigeon prep with legs fully engaged, torso upright.

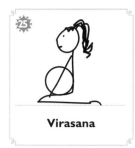

Virasana

Then with slight upper backbend (or supta with block behind back, first trimester only).

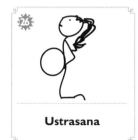

Ustrasana

With slight upper backbend or hands to heels (if comfortable).

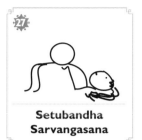

Setubandha Sarvangasana

Gentle lift of hips if comfortable. 3x. Rest on left side in between.

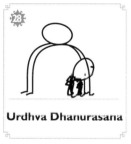

Urdhva Dhanurasana

If comfortable.

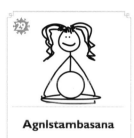

Agnistambasana

Keep feet active.

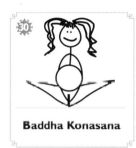

Baddha Konasana

Feet apart to fold forward.

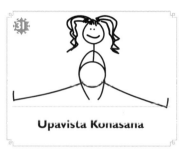

Upavista Konasana

Fold down middle.

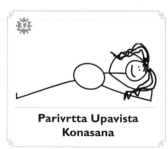

Parivrtta Upavista Konasana

Place the top hand behind the base of the skull and the bottom hand on the floor.

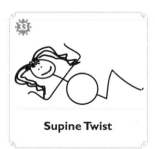

Supine Twist

Knees bent away from belly.

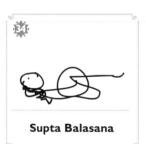

Supta Balasana

Lift head above heart after 4th month.

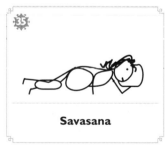

Savasana

With props on left side and between legs.

Restorative Sequence

Prenatal restorative postures encourage deep relaxation and stress relief, which support a pregnant woman in maintaining optimal health and avoiding injury and illness. If any of the poses feel uncomfortable, a pregnant woman should discontinue practicing them and try again another day. (Judith Lasater's book *Relax and Renew* is a great resource for restorative pose set ups.)

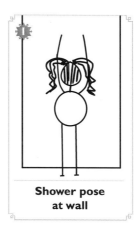

Shower pose at wall

(1-2 minutes): Facing the wall with arms stretched up, hands on wall.

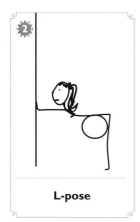

L-pose

(1-2 minutes): Relieves tension in back muscles, moves uterus up and forward out of pelvis, moves fetus away from nerves on back side of body, which may relieve spinal nerve pain.

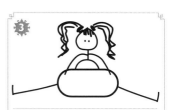

Upavista Konasana using a folding chair or several bolsters

(3-5 minutes): Soothes nervous system, releases hamstrings, quiets mind, relieves headaches and insomnia.

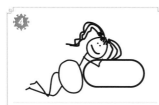

Reclining Gentle Twists with bolster

(30 seconds-2 minutes per side): Relieves stress on back muscles, stretches intercostal muscles between ribs, which may aid in breathing.

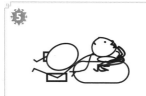

Supported Supta Baddha Konasana

(3-5 minutes): Deeper hip opener, benefits digestion and elimination, helps constipation, helps nasal congestion.

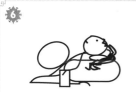

Supported Supta Virasana

(3-5 minutes): Helps relieve fatigue in legs, reduce swelling and varicose veins, relieves indigestion and nausea.

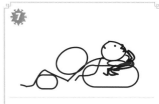

Supported Reclining Pose

(5 minutes): Calms nervous system, enhances breathing, reduces general fatigue, aids digestion and elimination.

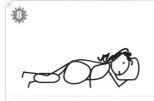

Supported Savasana on Left Side

(5-20 minutes): Relieves fatigue, nourishes baby with blood and oxygen, reduces high blood pressure.

Nausea Sequence

When it comes to nausea, take it slow and day to day. Stay longer in the poses that feel good and skip the ones that don't.

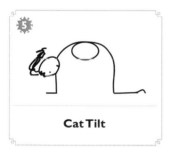

Child's Pose

5 gentle breaths.

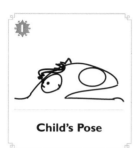

Vajrasana Ujjayi

Sit on tops of feet or blanket. Breathe 5 slow breaths.

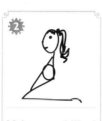

Virasana Nadi Shodhana

1 minute. Alternate nostril breathing, do not hold breath.

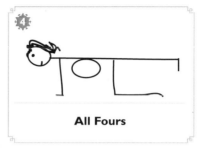

All Fours

One leg back at a time. 5 full breaths.

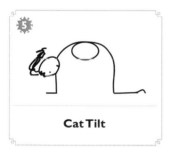

Cat Tilt

3x. Gentle movement in spine. Keep spine neutral on inhalation.

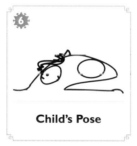

Child's Pose

5 gentle breaths.

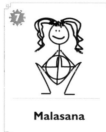

Malasana

30 seconds.

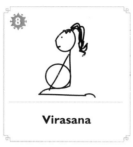

Virasana

Use block or blanket if needed. Root thighs.

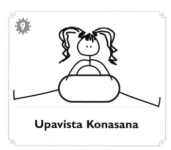

Upavista Konasana

30 seconds. Fold forward if possible, rest on bolster.

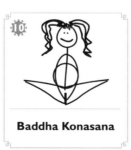

Baddha Konasana

30 seconds.

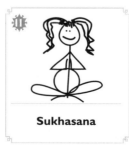

Sukhasana

5 full breaths.

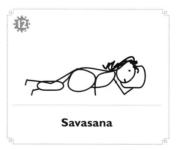

Savasana

With props on left side and between legs.

Infertility Sequence (Mixed Level)

This sequence should be done focusing on stretching the legs and rooting the femurs. New students should be with a teacher to ensure alignment.

1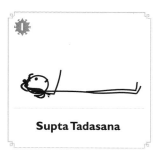

Supta Tadasana

Keep curve in lower back. Arms overhead (up and down) with breath.

2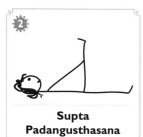

Supta Padangusthasana

Bottom leg rooted to floor, top leg straight up. Use strap if needed.

3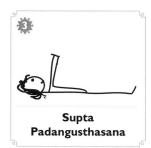

Supta Padangusthasana

Bend top knee towards floor.

4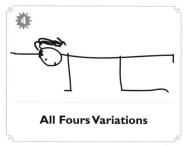

All Fours Variations

Balancing opposite arm/leg.

5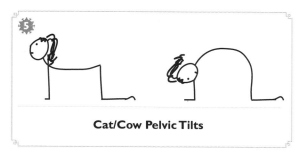

Cat/Cow Pelvic Tilts

5x. Link breath with movement.

6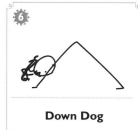

Down Dog

7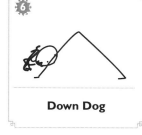

Uttanasana

With hands elevated on blocks if needed, root thighs back.

8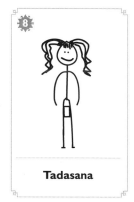

Tadasana

With block between upper inner thighs.

9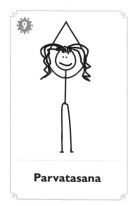

Parvatasana

Arms overhead. Root thighs back.

10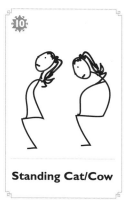

Standing Cat/Cow

Pelvic tilts.

11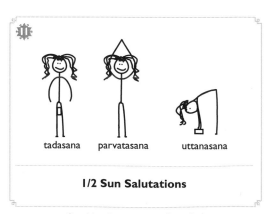

tadasana   parvatasana   uttanasana

1/2 Sun Salutations

3x. Hands on blocks if needed.

...continued on next page

Infertility Sequence (Mixed Level)

...continued from page 72

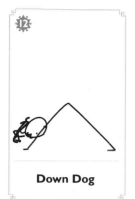

12

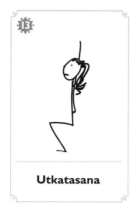

13

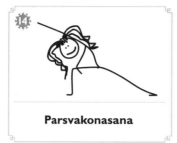

Parsvakonasana

Engage legs. Move inner thighs and sitting bones back.

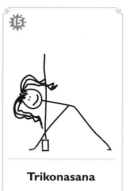

15

Down Dog

Utkatasana

Trikonasana

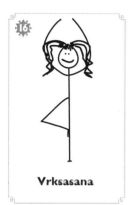

16

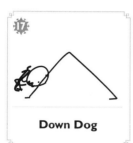

17

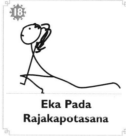

18

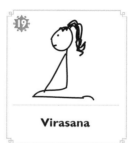

19

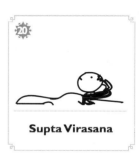

20

Vrksasana

Down Dog

Eka Pada Rajakapotasana

Keep inner thighs engaged.

Virasana

Use block or blanket if needed.

Supta Virasana

If comfortable.

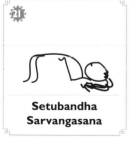

21

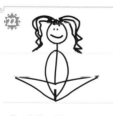

22

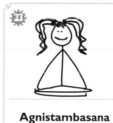

23

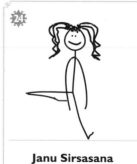
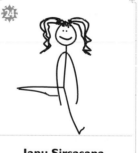

24

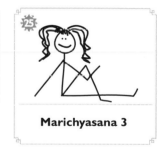

25

Setubandha Sarvangasana

Keep thighs parallel.

Baddha Konasana

Sit on blanket if needed.

Agnistambasana

Fold forward if possible.

Janu Sirsasana

Marichyasana 3

Ground foundation on the side you are turning towards.

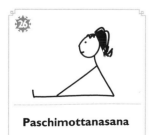

26

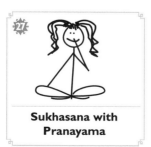

27

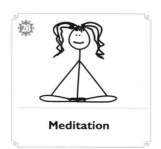

28

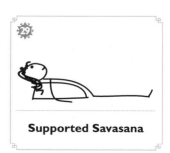

29

Paschimottanasana

Legs straight, root femurs.

Sukhasana with Pranayama

Alternate nostril breathing.

Meditation

Sit on blanket.

Supported Savasana

Allow pelvis and thighs to settle.

PRENATAL YOGA SYLLABUS OF ASANAS

The following is a list of yoga postures that can be practiced safely during pregnancy — with the help of a qualified teacher to ensure proper alignment. All poses should be modified according to the level of practitioner and the trimester. Please make sure props are on hand, in particular blocks, blankets, and straps. Students new to yoga should avoid deep backbends, inversions, and any pose that does not feel appropriate. Advanced practitioners may want to add to this syllabus, keeping in mind the earlier section on what to avoid and be cautious of (see page 31).

STANDING POSES

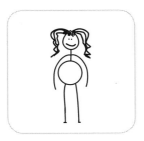

Tadasana
(mountain pose)

Parvatasana
(mountain pose with arms overhead)

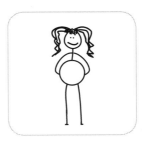

Tadasana Variation
(mountain pose with hands clasped behind back)

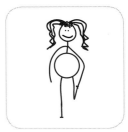

Standing Thigh Stretch

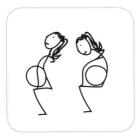

Standing Cat/Cow

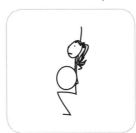

Utkatasana
(chair pose)

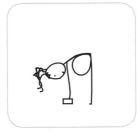

Uttanasana
(standing forward bend pose)

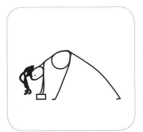

Parsvottanasana
(pyramid pose)

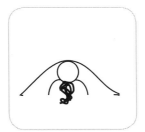

Prasarita Padottanasana
(wide-legged standing forward bend)

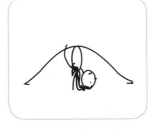

Parivrtta Prasarita Padottanasana
(twisting wide-legged standing forward bend)

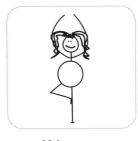

Vrksasana
(tree pose)

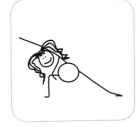

Parsvakonasana
(extended side angle pose)

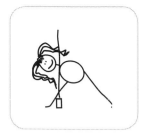

Trikonasana
(triangle pose)

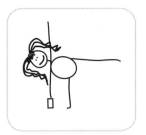

Ardha Chandrasana
(half moon pose)

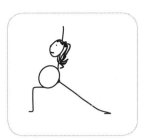

Virabhadrasana I
(warrior one pose)

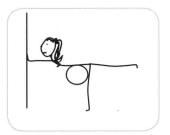

Virabhadrasana 3
(warrior three pose)

SITTING POSES, FORWARD BENDS, AND HIP OPENERS

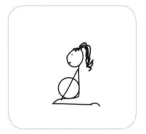

Virasana
(hero pose)

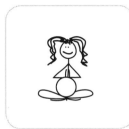

Sukhasana
(easy pose)

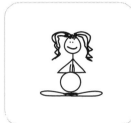

Siddhasana
(accomplished pose)

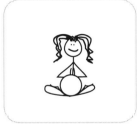

Padmasana
(lotus pose)

Baddha Konasana
(cobbler's pose)

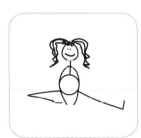

Janu Sirsasana
(modified
head to knee pose)

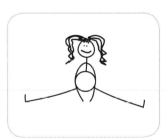

Upavista Konasana
(seated wide-angle
forward bend pose)

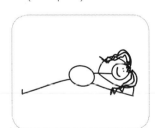

Parivrtta Upavista Konasana
(revolved seated wide-angle
forward bend pose)

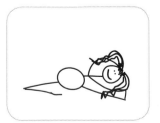

Parivrtta Janu Sirsasana
(modified revolved head
to knee pose)

Agnistambasana
(firelog pose)

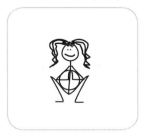

Malasana
(garland pose)

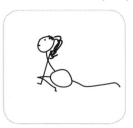

**Eka Pada
Rajakapotasana Prep**
(pigeon prep pose)

INVERSIONS AND HAND BALANCINGS

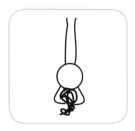

Sirsasana
(headstand pose)

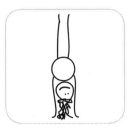

**Adho Mukha
Vrksasana**
(handstand pose)

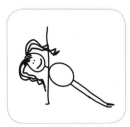

Vasisthasana
(side plank pose)

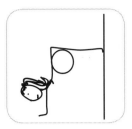

Inverted L-Pose

BACKBENDS

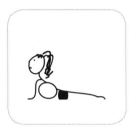

Bhujangasana
(cobra pose
with bolster)

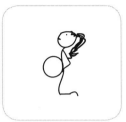

Ustrasana
(camel pose)

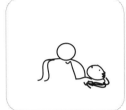

**Setubandha
Sarvangasana**
(bridge pose)

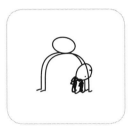

Urdhva Dhanurasana
(upward facing
bow pose)

MISCELLANEOUS

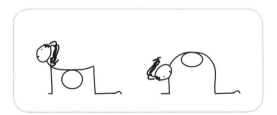

Cat/Cow Pelvic Tilts

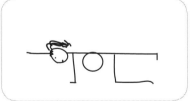

All Fours Variations
(balancing opposite arm/leg)

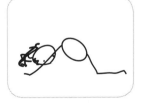

**Adho Mukha
Svanasana Prep**
(quarter dog)

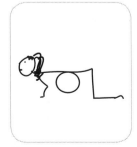

Chaturanga Push-ups
(four-limbed staff pose)

**Adho Mukha
Svanasana**
(down dog)

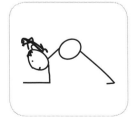

**Pinca Mayurasana
Prep**
(dolphin)

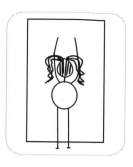

**Shower Pose
at Wall**

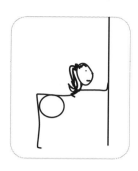

L-Pose

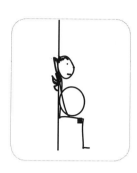

Wall Squat

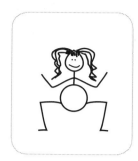

Goddess Pose

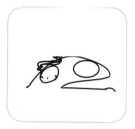

Balasana
(child's pose)

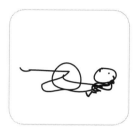

Supine Twist

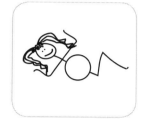

Supta Balasana
(reclined child's pose)

RESTORATIVES

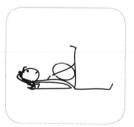

**Supta
Padangusthasana**
(reclined thigh-rooting
yoga pose)

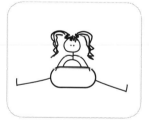

**Savasana
with Bolster**
(supported corpse pose)

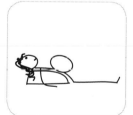

**Upavista Konasana using
Several Bolsters**
(supported wide-angle
forward bend pose)

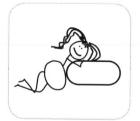

**Reclining Gentle Twists
with Bolster**

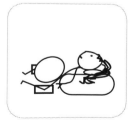

**Supported Supta
Baddha Konasana**
(reclined cobbler's pose)

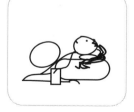

**Supported Supta
Virasana**
(reclined hero pose)

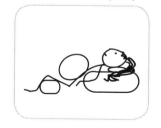

**Supported
Reclining Pose**

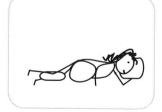

**Supported Savasana
on Left Side**
(reclined corpse pose)

ADDITIONAL RESOURCES

SUGGESTED READING LIST

Balaskas, Janet. Active Birth: *The New Approach to Giving Birth Naturally*, The Harvard Common Press, 1992.

Balaskas, Janet. *Preparing for Birth with Yoga: Empowering and Effective Exercise for Pregnancy and Childbirth*, Thorsons, 2003.

Balaskas, Janet and Yehudi Gordon. *The Encyclopedia of Pregnancy and Birth*: *A Complete Self Help Guide to Active Birth and Early Parenthood, Including an A-Z of Modern Obstetrics*, Little, Brown Book Group, 1989.

Bradley, Robert. *Husband-Coached Childbirth: The Bradley Method of Natural Childbirth*, Bantam, 2008.

Calais-Germain, Blandine. *The Female Pelvis: Anatomy and Exercises*, Eastland Press Inc., 2003.

England, Pam and Rob Horowitz, Ph.D. *Birthing from Within: An Extra-Ordinary Guide to Childbirth Preparation*, Partera Press, 1998.

Fawcett, Margaret. *Aromatherapy for Pregnancy and Childbirth*, Element Books, 1993.

Friend, John. *Anusara Yoga Teacher Training Manual*, Anusara Press, 2008.

Gaskin, Ina May. *Ina May's Guide to Childbirth*, Bantam, 2003.

Gerber, Magda. *Dear Parent: Caring for Infants with Respect*, Resources for Infant Educators, 2003.

Gordon, Jay. *Listening to Your Baby: A New Approach to Parenting Your Newborn,* The Berkley Publishing Group, 2002.

Harris, A. Christine Ph.D. *The Pregnancy Journal: A Day-to-Day Guide to a Healthy and Happy Pregnancy*, Chronicle Books, 2005.

Heller, Sharon Ph.D. *The Vital Touch: How Intimate Contact With Your Baby Leads to Happier, Healthier Development*, Holt Paperbacks, 1997.

Khalsa, Gurmukh Kaur. *Bountiful, Beautiful, Blissful: Experience the Natural Power of Pregnancy and Birth with Kundalini Yoga and Meditation*, St Martin's Griffin, 2004.

Lasater, Judith Ph.D. *Relax and Renew: Restful Yoga for Stressful Times*, Rodmell Press, 1995.

Leboyer, Frederick. *Birth Without Violence*, Healing Arts Press, 2009.

Mayo Clinic. *Mayo Clinic Complete Book of Pregnancy and Baby's First Year*, William Morrow, 1994.

McCall, Timothy. *Yoga as Medicine: The Yogic Prescription for Health and Healing*, Bantam, 2007.

Mongan, Marie F. *HypnoBirthing, The Mongan Method: A Natural Approach to a Safe, Easier, More Comfortable Birthing*, Health Communications, Inc., 2005.

Pearce, Joseph Chilton. *Magical Child*, Plume, 1992.

Sears, Martha RN and William Sears M.D. *The Baby Book: Everything You Need to Know About Your Baby from Birth to Age Two*, Little, Brown and Company, 2003.

Sears, Martha RN, William Sears M.D. and Linda Hughey Holt. *The Pregnancy Book*, Little, Brown & Company, 1997.

Simkin, Penny. *The Birth Partner: Everything You Need to Know to Help a Woman Through Childbirth*, Harvard Common Press, 2007.

Small, Meredith F. *Our Babies, Ourselves: How Biology and Culture Shape the Way We Parent*, Anchor, 1999.

Verny, Thomas M.D. and John Kelly. *The Secret Life of the Unborn Child: How You Can Prepare Your Baby for a Happy, Healthy Life*, Dell, 1982.

Weed, Susan. *Wise Woman Herbal: The Childbearing Year*, Ash Tree Publishing, 1985.

ONLINE RESOURCES
Anusara yoga — to learn more about Anusara yoga:

anusara.com

sueelkind.com

Birth:

birthintobeing.com

birthpsychology.com

babyfriendlyusa.org

Breastfeeding — for more information or difficulty:

llli.org (La Leche League)

kellymom.com

Breech presentation — and for information about optimal fetal positioning:

spinningbabies.com

Cesarean — information on c-sections:

ican-online.org

mayoclinic.com

Circumcision

nocirc.org

Doula — to learn more or locate one in your area:

dona.org

fromwombtoworld.com

Essential oils:

originalswissaromatics.com

oshadhiusa.com

Online magazines:

fitpregnancy.com

mothering.com

Parenting — from conception through the childhood years:

askdrsears.com

drjaygordon.com

Postpartum:

postpartum.net

Preconception:

babycenter.com

foresight-preconception.org.uk

Pregnancy information:

americanpregnancy.org

childbirth.org

cordbloodeducationcenter.com

pregnancy.about.com

pregnancyweekly.com

prenatalkula.com

motherandchildhealth.com

socalbirth.com

Prenatal nutrition — for information on essential nutrients and harmful foods:

mayoclinic.com

Prenatal yoga routine and interview with Sue Elkind:

fitpregnancy.com/yourpregnancy/prenatal_workout/the-power-of-yoga-40729172.html

Crunch Yoga Mama - prenatal yoga video(2000) - Sue Elkind — amazon.com

Vaccinations:

nvic.org

Waterbirths:

waterbirthsolutions.com

*"And then the time came,
when the risk it took to remain tight in a bud,
was more painful than
the risk it took to bloom"*
— Anais Nin

I would like to thank my beloved teacher John Friend for illuminating my life with these great teachings of Anusara yoga. I would also like to thank the following teachers, guides, and friends for inspiring me to listen to my heart and see this book through from conception to birth: Dr. Mae Sakharov, Barbara Benedict, Dana Covello, Gina Rubel, Kim Kemper, Douglas Brooks, Naime Jezzeny, and of course, my beautiful boys Luca and Milo.